How
Behavioral
Optometry
Can Unlock Your
Child's Potential

How
Behavioral Optometry
Can Unlock Your Child's Potential

Identifying and Overcoming Blocks
to Concentration, Self-Esteem and
School Success with Vision Therapy

Joel H. Warshowsky

Jessica Kingsley *Publishers*
London and Philadelphia

First published in 2012
by Jessica Kingsley Publishers
116 Pentonville Road
London N1 9JB, UK
and
400 Market Street, Suite 400
Philadelphia, PA 19106, USA

www.jkp.com

Library of Congress Cataloging in Publication Data
Warshowsky, Joel H.
How behavioral optometry can unlock your child's potential : identifying and
overcoming blocks to concentration, self-esteem and school success with
vision therapy / Joel H. Warshowsky.
p. cm.
Includes bibliographical references and index.
ISBN 978-1-84905-881-0 (alk. paper)
1. Behavioral optometry. 2. Visual training. 3. Vision disorders in
children. I. Title.
RE48.2.C5W37 2012
615.8'2--dc23
2011031445

British Library Cataloguing in Publication Data
A CIP catalogue record for this book is available from the British Library

ISBN 978 1 84905 881 0
eISBN 978 0 85700 617 2

Printed and bound in the United States

Dedicated to the enhancement of vision its impact
on learning and the development of self

Contents

PART III SPECIFIC VISION PROBLEMS AND BEHAVIORAL OPTOMETRIC INTERVENTIONS

Acknowledgments

As I look into my past, I find myself moving through the corridors of my mind as if I were opening up this old family chest high up in the attic. Upon opening the chest, I find an old newspaper clipping yellowed and torn with age, yet the writing remains as it had originally been. The words are as clear as they were when they were freshly typed. I, like so many of us, have struggled to be where I am today. But, just as clear as those typed letters and words on that dingy newspaper clipping, I clearly know those individuals who stood by me, letting me know that I could when many were saying that I could not. This book would not have been written if it were not for these individuals.

Let me begin with those optometrists whom I've learned so much from either through personal interaction or their written material. They have been a platform upon which I've been able to stand, helping me to believe in myself so that I would be able to practice my profession in the best way I thought possible: Norman Haffner, A.M. Skeffington, Nathan Flax, Irwin Suchoff, Micky Weinstein, Al Rappaport, Elliot Forest, Dan Wolf, Leonard Werner, Ed Johnston, Marty Birnbaum, Harold Solan, Sid Groffman, Allen Cohen, Arnie Sherman, Jacob Lieberman, Al Sutton, Amiel Francke, Robert A. Kraskin, Larry MacDonald, Bruce Wolff, Dick Appell,

Gerry Getman, John Streff, Andrea Thau, Carl Gruning, David Fitzgerald, Jack Richman, Ken Cuiffreda, Paul Harris, Glen Steele, and Rochelle Mozlin. I am able to write this book, and practice my profession because of those practitioners who in the past created and practiced the core philosophy that behavioural optometry now represents. Unlike medicine, our history is young, enabling our present thinking to go back to its core values. Throughout this book I make reference to first and second generation behavioural optometrists in order to show respect to those individuals whose shoulders upon whom we presently stand.

There have been many occupational therapists (OTs) and physical therapists (PTs) who have taught me about body dynamics critically important in the development of vision and visions ability to process information. Then there were those who went further in developing the co-joined therapy concept that exists today: Laurie Kalb, Phyllis Gordon, Sheila Allen, Marie Leo, Sylvia Hershkowitz, Susan Oetting, Carrie Strauch, Celeste Furmansky, Joanne Swenson, Rivka Vann, Maryann Martin, Dorothy Fox, Lorraine Aloysio, and Debbie Fuggini.

To the social workers, psychologists, and psychiatrists who taught me the distinct relation between vision and one's development of self, I will be forever grateful. Then there were those who taught me that understanding my own sense of self was critically essential to understanding my patient: Maureen O'Connor, Louis Schneider, Florence Springer, Michael Singer, and Michael Leiman.

To all the interns and residents whom I've had the pleasure to work with all of these years, you've taught me how to learn.

Then there are people throughout my life and career who stood by me with a clear sense of purpose, desire, and belief that their support for me would always be there. Bruchie Langsam always made this clear.

I wish to gratefully acknowledge the contribution of Dr. Charles Koch, retired educator, for helping to make my words "reader friendly."

My practice became the place where most of my clinical triumph evolved. If it were not for my staff, I would not have been able to make the changes in the lives of children in the way that I have. I am especially grateful to those who manage my offices: Annette Scorcia and Irene Vitale.

To my children, Justin and Jaime, who have always been for me a light that shines in so many places, opening my eyes to what is real and to what is truly important. Your strength, trust, and love have often been all that I needed to get through the hard times and have shown me how to enjoy the good times.

And to that one person who lets me know all that is good in me and all that I am capable of becoming: my beautiful, inside and out, wife Nicole. Without her strength of conviction, her ceaseless encouragement, her ability to know what is true from what is not true, and her boundless love, I could not have completed this book. She is the one who brings light to where it may not have been before.

Finally, I am truly grateful to all those people at Jessica Kingsley Publishers, namely Lisa Clark, Lucy Buckroyd, Emily McClave, and Claire Cooper, who have taken on this project as their own.

Preface

In the song "Empty Garden (Hey Hey Johnny)", Elton John calls out to his friend Johnny to come out and play.

Unlike Elton John's eulogy to John Lennon, the Johnny I'm talking about will be able to come out and play, but maybe not today. You see, Johnny, who just began third grade, is not able to get his homework done in time to play with his friends today.

As we all know, playtime is a special time during which children sense all that life can be. For them it's the time to fantasize and to dream the dreams that make them special. It's a time full of all the stuff that makes them children. For all the Johnnies who can't have this special time, there grows a feeling of despair and hopelessness. How very sad for our Johnny, for it is his dreams of today that will shape so many of his tomorrows.

Many children have trouble finishing their homework. They simply have difficulty in school and as a result become frustrated. Unfortunately, their frustrations grow most often after they have been somewhat successful in earlier grades. For our Johnny, that would have been first and second grade, and yes, even kindergarten.

Very often children like Johnny, perhaps even your son or daughter, have vision problems that are the cause of their difficulties. And no amount of extra help or even special tutoring will address the cause of those difficulties.

For many children, difficulties in school are the result of an eye muscle imbalance that limits how long they can look at something. Think about that. If your youngster has difficulty looking at something, anything—say words on a printed page—for any length of time, is it any wonder that he or she is having difficulty with school work, difficulty reading?

Ah but you say, he did so well last year, perhaps it is the teacher he has this year. Before we look for an obscure culprit, let's consider a potential cause over which he presently has no control. And, if that cause is an eye muscle imbalance, then the more he tries to overcome his difficulty, with increased study, or extra help, or even tutoring, the more he will add to his already vexing problem.

Consider the following—in reading, the smaller the print and the more information available, the harder it is to look, to see, and to understand. Second and third grade is a typical time for children to begin having difficulty because that is when the print in their books becomes smaller and reading content becomes more involved. Skills that develop learning to read now have to become skills to develop reading to learn. Many of these youngsters get what can only be called a *dazed* look about them. It's as if they are staring right past you. What they are doing is relaxing their eyes just as you might do at the end of the day. They seem to be daydreaming but what they are really doing is trying to reduce the eyestrain experienced throughout that day.

Eyestrain is the result of two sets of eye muscles designed to work together but not working together. One muscle system controls focus for clarity while the other controls the function of seeing single and not double. Vision difficulties can involve either of these systems alone or the function of the two systems working together. Classical symptoms resulting from eyestrain are excessive rubbing of one's eyes, headaches and eye pain typically after near visual activities, double vision at times, blurred vision, missing or substituting words while reading, difficulty finishing school work, and—the most common symptom—consistent loss of place and/or skipping of lines. And then there are those youngsters without any apparent symptoms at all. They are the children who do not display symptoms simply because they avoid any situation that calls for them to read or write for any considerable length of time.

Vision therapy is the treatment for these kinds of problems as well as other vision problems discussed in this book. The success of vision therapy, regardless of the age of the patient, depends on the motivation of the team involved in the treatment. The team includes three key elements: the patient, the parents, and the behavioral optometrist. (Note: if the patient is an adult, then the parent is almost never a part of the team.) If the condition is recent and academic delays have not yet occurred, the procedure is actually quite simple and almost always results in complete remediation. When the condition is of a long-standing nature, frustration ensues. Academic and/or emotional concerns often become secondary problems that need to be addressed along with the visual ones. Understandably, the more involved the situation, the more involved the treatment. When vision is not the only concern, the team must include appropriate additional professionals. Therefore, if academics are an issue, special education professionals may be called in. Social workers and psychologists may be consulted if emotional and/or psychological concerns are presented. Physical and occupational therapists for sensory motor conditions and speech pathologists for speech and language issues may be needed to complete the team.

Johnny, and maybe your son or daughter, must be free to play with all the other children today. They, in fact all children, must be able to imagine and fantasize so that their dreams of today become society's realities of tomorrow. John Lennon won't be able to play with us today, but Johnny or your Justin and Jaime can. John Lennon's dreams will be with us forever. Your child's dreams must also be given the chance to be nurtured and allowed to survive in order to be with us forever as well. This book will do exactly that: it will give your child his or her chance.

My Vision for This Book

The visual, motor, and/or auditory dysfunctions children face are but one obstacle to their success. The greater obstacle, however, is misunderstanding what they encounter as a result of their dysfunction. They are told that they are wrong. They are told that they are bad. They are even told that they are stupid. Not always in so many words, but the message is nevertheless clear: they are the problem. And as a result of that message, spoken or implied, the harm is done: self-image is severely damaged. Their sense of failure becomes all-pervasive. They simply do not feel safe and they do not have the inner resources to become safe on their own. On top of the perceptual challenges they face, they must also face the challenges of rejection, of pain, and of loneliness. I wrote this book because no child should have to face all of these challenges at the same time. We as parents and as professionals have a responsibility to them, to meet them where they are, to see the world through their eyes, and to guide them to a new and healthier understanding of their full potential and value in this world. They need our help.

Some get help: psychotherapy, occupational therapy, physical therapy, speech and language therapy, as well as special education. Many show improvement as a result, but the root cause of their problem goes untreated if the root is vision. When symptoms of that root and not causes are treated, an unfortunate result is that the child does not become visually independent, and does not learn to self-remediate in a variety of areas. It's not uncommon to hear from other therapists that, although they have taken a child as far as they can, other significant problems remain. This is not a criticism of other forms of therapy; it is to say, however, that not all forms of therapy succeed in making a child failure free across a wide spectrum of tasks and within a wide range of circumstances. That, however, is the aim of behavioral optometry's vision therapy.

What do I mean by failure free? By failure free, I mean children free from visual limitations that would otherwise create a situation of failure if left to their typical course. I mean children who no longer define themselves by their visual limitations. I mean children who have developed a new sense of self through the visual realm with confidence and a new sense of self-fortitude that will potentially carry forward into every aspect of their life. The methods and philosophy contained in this book do just that: we take children to a place where they no longer define themselves as a failure, but, rather, define themselves as a success.

So how do we do that? Although we possess five senses, we principally learn how to function within our environment through three senses: visual, auditory, and motor. Approximately 80 percent of information processed is visual. Vision, as the primary interfacing sense, acts in such a way that correcting one element of a complex system will have profound effects throughout the system.

The process of training children to reframe their visual relationship with the world is not only about vision. It is about utilizing vision to reframe the relationship between children's inner reality and their external reality. Vision is merely the vehicle, the classroom, the training ground. The true benefits accrue when a child, perhaps your son or daughter, takes what he or she has achieved in the safe and nurturing environment of therapy and applies it to the outside world. It is then that children's entire sense of who they are and what they are capable of, has been modified for the better. And that modification has the potential to last a lifetime.

There are many people who do not know that there exists a specialized field in optometry called behavioral optometry. And then there are those who have heard of behavioral optometry but are not aware of its significance. This book has been written to bring light to where there may be none.

The book will answer the question: What is behavioral optometry all about, and how will it help my child become his or her ultimate true self? Through it I will unlock the mystery of the tools, techniques, and philosophy used by behavioral optometrists to achieve that goal. More than that, I will show how correction of misperception can actually result in greater than expected benefits, benefits well beyond the visual realm and into the realm of self-awareness. It is my steadfast belief, having over 35 years of experience, that these techniques based on a time-measured philosophy, can help a child—your child perhaps—achieve a stronger and healthier sense of self, one that will better connect him or her to the world in which he or she will live for a lifetime.

About me

My 35-year path began at the SUNY State College of Optometry. Before I got into this profession, I chose dentistry. I actually took the dental school entrance exam twice. All was fine except for the spatial relationship component of the test. I failed miserably. The handwriting was clearly written on the wall: *Joel, you won't make it in dentistry!* What my choices then were seemed to evolve into two somewhat related fields, podiatry or optometry. In as much as contact lenses had an appeal that toenail clippers lacked, optometry it was!

Soon I found myself immersed in the specialized area of contact lenses. Any thoughts of visual therapy were far from my mind. One day I found myself in need of information on accommodative esotropia (a crossed eye), a condition one of my patients had. As a result I met with Nathan Flax, my supervisor and chief of the vision therapy service. I clearly didn't know how to evaluate and/or treat this condition and Dr. Flax let me know with no uncertainty that I didn't have a clue.

Through Dr. Flax's efforts, I began to see the effect vision therapy could have on my patients. The changes were as direct and efficacious as the modifications I was making with hard contact lenses. Further, I soon became fascinated with the idea that not only could I affect patients' skills in such a consistent, reliable, and valid way, but I could also actually affect the way they felt about themselves. I approached my fourth year with my sights set on the vision training residency.

Up until that time, SUNY students had not been accepted into that program. At the end of my fourth year, I was accepted as the first SUNY professional in just the third SUNY Vision Therapy Residency Program. I was elated on hearing about my acceptance. But in the next moment I felt dejection and even panic. I realized that, if I were to see challenging therapy patients, I would naturally want to refer him to one of my own professors. Even more upsetting was the thought that patients might not even want to see me in the first place when they could go to whom I considered were the best in the field.

It was in that moment, however, that I came to a life-changing realization. Patients would come to me because I had something no one else had. That something was the essence of my own self, that inner understanding of who I am and why I exist. It was in that moment that I realized that my quest in vision therapy would serve to define me. It would define who I was as a person and who I would be as a vision therapist.

That moment of inner peace and confidence came, I am certain, from a place deep within. It all started, I believe, when I was 12 years old. I had just received my junior high school report card and was close to failing all my subjects. That didn't surprise me; after all, I had always suffered from reading and learning problems. In hindsight, failing the spatial relations section on the dental entrance exam turned out to be one of my old nemeses causing me to fail. Sadly, there didn't seem to be anyone who recognized the ability that was locked up within me. Even sadder was that it seemed to me that everyone—and I mean everyone—thought that these problems actually defined who I was: an unsuccessful kid.

It was then that I came to realize that, if I were to succeed in life, it—whatever that "it" was—would have to come from within me. The thoughts and feelings that came from that insight let me know that I could be whatever I chose to be. I had discovered that the choice was solely mine.

When I began my own practice, I became aware that my own struggles as a child truly led me to my profession and to the approaches I now use. Not only do I remember but I am still able to get in touch with those old feelings. It is because of those feelings that I am motivated to help my young patients find that same inner strength that I was able to find. I found that I could help children find their true selves. This is the core within me and this is what I am able to offer in my therapeutic treatment programs. When I treat a child, I am very much aware that within that child is a lovable, capable, and marvelously powerful being. I know that that's what I was looking for as a child. All everyone saw were the problems I presented. I never enjoyed the benefits of anyone seeing the "true me", of knowing the 'true me' of reacting to the "true me." I am convinced that all children who become aware of their "true self" will be able to reach their full potential and emerge as the powerful being they were meant to be. Self-awareness alone is often all that's necessary to begin a youngster's life-changing process. It is when self-awareness takes place that remediation begins. This book is all about a significant and powerful way to sensitize a child's spirit and enable the child's true self to emerge, and that emergence is through vision.

But what is vision really all about and what is its purpose?

Alexander Luria's global theory of brain function is a philosophy that explores the brain as programmable, dynamic and active. He presented the brain as an efficient and adaptive system geared for evolution and change, ceaselessly adapting to the needs of the organism. Its need above all is to construct a coherent self and world.

The ultimate purpose of vision is to create such an awareness of a real symmetrical space world. That awareness potentially translates into an awareness of self. Awareness of one's body in space is the foundation. Efficient acquiring and processing of visual information requires one to initially develop a stable internal representation of the 3-D structure of one's body in relation to one's environmental space world. Weinstein, second generation behavioral optometrist, states, "Thus, it appears that the organization of SELF, must precede the organization of space, and the latter refers to the former as its 'standard.'" (1967, p.1030)

It has long been understood that approximately 20 percent of light entering the eye affects lower brain stem function in support of the posturing mechanisms of one's body in space rather than to the higher centers of function. This postural mechanism plays a vital role in establishing an awareness of self, and that awareness is further developed through the additional control of one's eye coordination (convergence) and focus (accommodation). Robert Kraskin, first generation behavioral optometrist, highlights this understanding through the recognition of three levels of commitment required by the body as a product of information processing. The first level requires the body to be in balance with gravity (where am I?). The second level requires the accuracy of the two eyes to determine where objects are in relation to our body: eye coordination (where is it?). And third, once these two commitments are appreciated, a higher order of processing could be achieved: focus (what is it?). This illuminates the behavioral definition of vision: *the directing of action and deriving of meaning as a product of processing information triggered by a selected band of radiant energy (light).*

This overall concept is also embodied in the famous four-circle model of A.M. Skeffington, the father of behavioral optometry, a model which further defined vision and how it functions (Skeffington 1931). These four intersecting circles include the integrated processing of centering, identification, balance, and speech emerging into vision.

In behavioral optometry we say that vision is, as Skeffington explained, an emergent process. This process stems from the combined effect of centering (spatial awareness of objects in space in relation to self), identification (assessing meaning to objects focused upon), vestibular function (orientation of body in space, i.e. balance) and speech or language (ability to receive and express through words). From this one can begin to appreciate that vision is an involved and complicated process. Therefore, having good eyesight defined as 20/20 may in reality not be good vision at all.

> If one were to use the analogy of vision represented as a house, the aspect of the house that might be considered to represent 20/20 may be the door of the house while the rest of the house represents the totality of vision and one's subsequent visual perception and process.

Skeffington, states that vision is an external reflection of an internal neurological organization (2006, p.6). The essence of vision is not just physical or physiological. Vision is also an emotional, psychological, and neurological expression. What we see is actually the end result of a process that has already been initiated well before we actually see! Arnold Gesell, one of the most celebrated developmental pediatricians of our time, may have given us the best definitions of vision:

> Seeing is not a separate isolable function, it is profoundly integrated with the total action system of the child, his posture, manual skills and coordination, intelligence and even personality makeup. Indeed vision is so intimately identified with the whole child that we cannot understand its economy and its hygiene without investigating the whole child. (Gesell *et al.* p.10)

Therefore, behavioral optometry's vision therapy is a process of practicing procedures that result in patients becoming more physically, physiologically, mentally, and emotionally aware of themselves through the exploration of their vision and visual skills, which leads to a higher level of self-awareness. It is through this modification of one's vision and ultimately one's resultant perceptions that self-awareness is achieved. It is effective, efficient, and effortless visual function that creates a visual reality without visual distortion, making for a true self-perception. And that's the stage upon which awareness of one's true self is established and presented. This may be best summarized by Gerry Getman, first generation behavioral optometrist. He states:

> Parents, teachers and clinicians can set the stage, but only the child himself can act thereon. A child is taught nothing—he learns everything—and vision is the supreme mechanism a child possesses for the interpretation of his world. All other mechanisms discussed here are important for a "total child," but all are subservient to vision. (Getman 1993, p.124)

Children's attitude, motivation, discipline, and willpower determine their ability to reach the goal of effortless visual function. However, youngsters are often unaware that they are able to perform a visual activity with greater ease and efficiency and less effort. That is because they consider their usual and customary way of visually perceiving and interpreting as normal and constant. Unfortunately, they likewise experience their struggles as a self-reflection that then becomes the core upon which their sense of failure spirals downward.

Behavioral vision therapy considers vision in a way that lets children know they can develop effective, efficient, and effortless visual function with a resultant positive change in behavior and perception. This, in a very natural way, leads them to be able to resolve their own visual and associated behavioral dysfunctions. They are able to do this by being capable of going to the core of their visual dysfunction and remedying it.

Through vision therapy, I have become attuned to three levels of awareness necessary for a life-changing process to occur. These levels come from what is known as the cybernetic principles. They consist of the following:

- **Goal orientation:** Can I, the child, become aware of my problem? Can I recognize my goal?

- **Self-directed:** Do I, the youthful patient, desire to remediate the problem? Once aware, will I take the necessary steps to self-direct?

- **Self-correctable:** If I, the youngster, lose my way, will I be able to get back to my goal? Will I take the steps necessary to remediate? If I go off track, will I do what's necessary to self-correct?

The introduction of these three levels of awareness to a child has become the foundation and the framework of my practice. It has allowed me to discuss prognosis in a way that most frequently results in full remediation without regression. My goal is to establish within each child an insight that I first learned from one of my mentors, Marty Birnbaum, second generational behavioral optometrist. He stated that the ultimate success in therapy comes about when a child can actually function as their own therapist.

When this is established, what follows is truly beautiful to behold. Children reach a level of self-discovery within the visual process that introduces them to a new-found freedom heretofore unknown. It is a freedom to know and to cherish their very own true essence of self and to know their unique and special connectedness to the world.

I have discovered my purpose in life. It is my drive to uncover my own inner person that has led me to practice the way that I do. And that way helps each and every child I treat uncover his or her own magical self. I let them know that they can, while everything else about them tells them that they can't.

PART I

UNDERSTANDING VISION IN CHILDREN

BACKGROUND AND BASICS

Chapter 1

Understanding the Effects of the "Failure Syndrome" in a Child

Within each of us is a lovable, marvelously powerful being, our true self. I believe that it is our true inner sense of vision, to a significant degree, that enables us to sensitize our own spirit enabling our hidden self to emerge. Children who are aware of their true selves emerge into the powerful beings they truly are and thus reach their full potential. What greater gift can we give children than to help them in this process if and when that help is needed?

Recognizing the failure syndrome

Difficulties arise, either cognitively or emotionally, when a child's hidden true self does not emerge. As children continuously fail at a particular task that prevents the development of a specific skill, they frequently come to believe that they are the problem rather than their inability to achieve success with the task. That is to say, these children frequently believe they are wrong, rather than that they merely did something incorrectly. This is what I call the "failure syndrome." With this belief of failure, a sense of inadequacy begins to take root. Sadly, this is often characterized by a child withdrawing and not even attempting tasks that were previously performed with success. These children appear to enter into what has been identified by noted psychologist John Bradshaw as "toxic shame...a false self" (p.vii). Once that false sense takes hold, children will not only withdraw from a task, but also often develop adaptive compensations that in actuality further limit and distort their interaction with the task. This, most unfortunately, can last a lifetime.

Here's a metaphor that may help clarify the development of the failure syndrome.

> Many office buildings have two ceilings: a true ceiling as well as a false drop ceiling. The true ceiling is the actual interior side of the roof. The drop ceiling, on the other hand, is positioned below the true ceiling. It is there for decorative purposes. It hides wires, ductwork, and other assorted unattractive things. A drop ceiling gives the viewer a sense that the ceiling is lower than it actually is.

Similarly, a child in a spiral of failure sees his or her potential as more like the drop ceiling, lower than the true ceiling, lower than it actually is. Each time a mistake is made, children view their ceiling as coming down lower. With each mistake, the ceiling becomes lower still. Self-esteem, self-worth, and self-confidence all diminish as the ceiling lowers. Eventually children learn not to risk taking a chance, so that the ceiling may come down still lower. They become caught up in a self-preserving response, which translates into a self-preserving all too limiting response. They stop trying because they do not want to risk being smothered by their ever lowering boundary, that ever lowering ceiling. They will seek escape from being crushed, sadly, never realizing that their ever lowering ceiling is but a false ceiling. In reality, it is a ceiling that they alone have created. What they need to be made to see is that there need be no escape from what in actuality is a ceiling of their own creation. What they need to be made to see, through intervention, is that they can remain engaged in all their present activities and, most importantly, that they can feel safe while doing so.

By now I suppose you're asking, "Dr. Warshowsky, how do you recognize this syndrome?" My answer is that it often presents itself as unmotivated or motivated. Unmotivated and dejected children may simply withdraw, become inattentive, and display a lack of focus and concentration. They often react behaviorally by getting out of their seat inappropriately, talking out of turn or acting as the class clown. They may exhibit a lack of gross motor coordination, a lack of awareness of body and position in space, or organizational insecurity, and they may fall or bump into objects within their environment. They may see double, or print may appear to jump or shift; they may lose their place, skip lines, substitute or omit words, and/or have a need to reread in order to better comprehend what they have just read. Some children in this spiral of failure may actually act out with anger in response to evaluation procedures exposing their fear associated with a disorganized strategy in reading and learning and in knowing themselves.

In contrast to unmotivated children, motivated children display symptoms such as, but not limited to, headaches, stomach aches, overall fatigue, eye pain, distance and/or near visual blur, and subsequent increases in nearsightedness (myopia), which will be discussed in Chapter 10. Typically they will not appear as unstable as the unmotivated child, yet they will often seem stressed, fatigued or labored while engaged in visually demanding activities. At times they can be characterized as anxious and even angry.

The response that children go through is typically dependent upon their behavioral, cognitive, emotional and psychological nature, and their subsequent modes of adaptation. In each presentation, symptoms displayed are either an external physical expression of inner strife or are related to the compensations children go through in order to create an internal/external balance. This is in response to an imbalance between their cognitive ability (their ability to succeed in what they think they should be able to achieve) and their actual ability to perform in their environment. In short, children entering the *failure syndrome* demonstrate, in their own way, a sense of being at risk. They appear to be tense and untrusting, and going backward in their life while all their friends are moving forward.

Another typical question I am asked is, What about well-balanced and well-adjusted children with visual dysfunction? Do they exist? I find that it is not common to encounter a child with visual dysfunction who has maintained a true sense of self. However, when the well-balanced child does present, it is always associated with loving, caring, nurturing parents, coupled with a supportive family environment that is not critical of the child's shortcomings. Such children are taught that they are not the problem limiting their success; rather, that they simply have difficulty with a particular task. Children with visual dysfunction, who have somehow maintained a true sense of self, can still have symptoms, and those symptoms may include academic ones (e.g., mistakes in reading) or physical ones (e.g., stress, headache, and eye pain). However, unquestionably, nurturing love and the confidence in our children can override the depressed feelings associated with the failure syndrome. Even though the dysfunction still needs to be addressed, I have found that such children move through the program more easily than those who are also challenged by difficulties in relationship or environment. They respond with greater ease to a self-directing, self-correcting, goal-oriented regimen. Recognize that children will most often present as some combination of these descriptions, usually with an emphasis on one.

Overcoming the failure syndrome

The obvious next question is how is it possible to break through to children struggling in this spiral of failure? How do we let them know that their perception of the dropped ceiling is false? How do we let them know that their true potential is not related to their failures, but rather that their true potential is only relative to the height of their aspirations? If they were able to break through the tiles of the false ceiling, the actual ceiling's real nature would be exposed. It is when the therapist creates the stage for a child to perceive the false ceiling for what it is that the child's false perception of self begins to shatter. It is then that the child begins to develop a true understanding of his or her own true potential.

Breaking through or, better still, eliminating the false ceiling begins with trust. An integral component of that trust comes with a change in a child's understanding and willingness to remove the false ceiling. Remediation is achieved through sensory motor technique, yet only through committed trust will children venture forth challenging their own sense of balance within space. And how do we create that trust? A.M. Skeffington stated that people who are unstable in their visual world are unstable in their ego. Recognition by the therapist, parent, and child of the association between the child's visual dysfunction and his or her lack of sense of self creates a stage upon which trust can be built. And as a result of the development of that trusting relationship between the child and therapist, remediation can potentially occur. Steps toward remediation are achieved through physical, physiological, and perceptual techniques utilized within the vision therapy program. Our goal is always to create therapeutic techniques systematically set up for all children to succeed. This is our entry card into their world.

What follows is a case that highlights a child with an internal/external struggle and how a trusting relationship was subsequently built to resolve his conflict.

A child presented at SUNY with visual acuities of 20/20 in the right eye and 20/40 in the left. The optometry intern evaluating the child on my behalf became perplexed while presenting this case to me. The vision in the child's left eye remained reduced even as the intern utilized the called-for prescriptive lens as part of his evaluation. Strangely, the left eye was still seeing at 20/40 vision with or without the proper therapeutic measures, and there was no other reason for the reduced vision.

As I entered the exam room, I saw this 9-year-old little boy sitting in the big examination chair, feet dangling above the floor, wondering what was to happen next. Intimidated and anxious, he seemed to be trying his best to face the situation bravely. As I sat down next to him, I placed my hand on his shoulder and spoke softly in a way that conveyed my desire to help him. I knew that I could, and I also knew that he wanted me to. Communicating this sense of mutual understanding is often intuitively conveyed, especially with children. While physical contact and tone are important, so are spoken words. So I said to him, "I know that you know that your two eyes are different." And then I paused. Continuing again I said, "And I know that you want me to know that." Again I paused. "I'm letting you know that I know." I again paused and then went on, "And now for me to help you I need you to tell me what you see." With that I re-measured his acuities. He was now reading at 20/20 with either eye.

What was happening was a case of a self-depressed visual system influenced by emotional imbalance. This child's problem was not necessarily his eye, which indeed had a slight visual defect. The root problem was his desperate need to be understood, to let others know what he already knew, namely that his left eye didn't perceive as his right did. In this need to have his external reality validated, he needed to make his sight defect worse. He was fearful that he would not be understood and he didn't have confidence that he would be able to communicate his deficiency effectively. But when I let him know that he had, in me, an external validation of his defect, he had no further need to amplify his problem, I listened and heard.

Who we see ourselves to be, and our resulting future reality, frequently come from how we see our inside self matched with our outside self. Jean Piaget, a noted learning theorist of the last century, stated that appropriate learning takes place when there is a match between what is within us (internal) and what is outside us (external). He called this concept "equilibrium" (Flavell 1996; Piaget and Inhelder 1966). The children we are discussing often present in a state of disequilibrium. Such children seek correction, but often ineffectively or inappropriately by protecting their inner perception at the expense of their external reality. When children are unsure about what they see outside of themselves, they have the option of making up what they think they should be seeing. They do this in order to create some sense of an internal/external balance. Their compensation develops in order to hide or cover up their sense of deficiency or inadequacy. Thus, they will limit their interaction with the object world and try to enhance their internally generated false sense of what they think is real. How often do we hear children add or delete from what they have read, heard, or experienced? Their reality is cognitive but falsely driven, trying to create what they think they should see. It is, by definition, false, or, at best, a self-generated projection of reality within which they try to exist. At the least, they fear their world.

Just as visual dysfunction can influence emotional balance, so too can insecurity or emotional imbalance result in a depressed visual system. It works both ways. This is illustrated by a 47-year-old female patient who came into my office for treatment of a visually related reading disability.

My diagnosis was that of an eye turning outward, or the patient's inability to turn her eyes inward, to converge (exotropic strabismus). She was aware of its occurrence at various times of the day but totally unaware of why it was occurring. Through probing conversation, I was able to make an association between her eyes turning outward and a long-standing depression. It was a case of emotional imbalance creating a depressed visual system. I was able to trace both the depression and the turning outward of her eye to a time when she was 4 years old. It was then that her mother developed a chronic debilitating emotional condition. When I spoke to her about how I perceived her situation, she was able to express her condition as obsessive circular thinking associated with her depression. Not surprising to me, her depression began to disappear as her convergence ability progressed. In a short time, she expressed her ability to visually focus as a way to turn her depression "off like a faucet." Presently, she has developed an awareness of her visual problem and has a goal orientation through visual therapy that has been able to achieve self-direction and self-correction. In practice, I often experience an association between acute and/or chronic emotional and/or psychological conditions and visual dysfunction. That was clearly the case here. When the patient learned to straighten her eyes, her depression diminished and increased again only when she allowed her eyes to turn out again. This awareness allowed her to achieve her own comfort level of remediation.

These two cases not only highlight the association between internal and external struggles within a patient, but also that the mechanism can operate in either direction. Both cases illustrate how internal strife can lie at the heart of a patient's difficulties. Stabilizing the external environment through visual techniques served to create the opportunity, the platform, for a balanced internal/external sense.

Building a relationship of trust

The challenge in treating children with these conditions is not just learning how to diagnose, treat, and manage visual dysfunction. There are wonderful texts that describe in detail how to accomplish these things. No, the challenge is in learning to approach dysfunction in a way that enables remediation rather than simply improving upon the condition. Remediation in this regard involves empowering children to trust in themselves, and to accept and understand themselves enough to ultimately self-correct their dysfunction. Full remediation is the goal because it is the only antidote to the false self-perception that children rely upon to self-preserve. Internal/external equilibrium is my goal, external remediation is my means.

Empowering children to trust and understand who they are and what their role is within a visual context is central to the remediation of their associated behavioral anomalies. This empowerment takes place when the clinician is willing and able to cross over an invisible clinical line and to develop a very personal therapeutic rapport with the patient. The willingness to seek out visual intimacy with patients is up to the individual clinician. This they must assess and decide for themselves. Most assuredly, it is not an invitation to disregard accepted and appropriate guidelines for personal interaction within the clinical setting. However, the mainstream of our profession concerns itself with merely getting an image onto the retina. Our true realm is not the world of muscles and optics. Rather, it is what is happening beyond that. It is what is happening deep within the child's inner world, and his or her ability to process the outer world with ease.

There is a Chinese proverb that says, "If you cannot find it in yourself, where will you go for it?" Each child, in fact each of us, can only receive from others what we have already seen and have thus created within ourselves. Importantly, any dysfunction that affects vision will, by its very nature, have an impact on how we see, and thus how we perceive and, ultimately, how we feel.

Now, here is the important part of the equation for it is the result. Children with visual disabilities are limited by what and how they see things, resulting in how they feel about themselves. Visual dysfunction, even minor ones, have a negative impact on self-image. Think about it: children—and subsequently adults—struggling with visual dysfunction are not aware that what they are viewing is in any way distorted, or in any way less than absolute. Then, when what to them under the pretext of reality is visually acted upon, it is no wonder self-doubt results. The more severe one's visual dysfunction, the greater the potential for visual distortion. Unfortunately, when this occurs, there is almost always a negative impact on self-image. Imagine living in a world not knowing what is real and what is illusion, as a result of misperception.

> Consider going into a fun house, with all the mirrors, in an amusement park. It's fun at first, but then all you want to do is escape. Our kids with visual dysfunction can't escape, they can't get out.

Sadly, individuals who are lacking in self-worth soon learn that making a mistake or doing something wrong means that they are the mistake or that they are what's wrong. When children reach this state, they begin to demonstrate a lack of awareness of their own internal personal identity. They assume roles and scripts given to them by significant others such as parents, teachers, or doctors. They receive mixed messages about what they see, or what they should be seeing, how they feel, or how they should be feeling. The end result of this self-manipulation is a lack of self-worth that often degenerates into a self-fulfilling prophecy of despair.

I believe that being on an emotional level with a child becomes the platform upon which vision connects from the heart. This is how I begin to work with young people to free them from their sense of despair. Let me explain. It is my belief that, in order for children to recognize errors in judgment, they must first feel a relationship in which there exists no fear or misgiving about what they do. They need to feel that, in the event that one of their perceptions is wrong, it is not they who are wrong. Rather, it is their perception that is inaccurate. It is the feelings that comes from the heart that give children the opportunity to trust, and it is their vision that gives them direction, a vehicle in which to proceed.

Trust in a relationship is the cornerstone upon which a child begins to develop a true sense of self. A vision therapy program incorporating tracking, focusing, and coordination skills are the tools upon which this cornerstone of reality of self can be built. These tools structure the way a child is led to develop a stable sense of self through a realized stable environment. This can only be recognized when the integral part of the relationship is trust between the doctor and child. The enhancement of tracking, focusing, and eye coordination skills directs, in a most natural way, the establishment of a sound stable perception. Once accomplished, the development of voluntary convergence—that is the ability to voluntarily turn one's eyes inward—results in a feeling of elation, a sense of well-being. This is because the child is now able to make purposeful visual judgments resulting in accurate visual perceptions. Ultimately, the ability to effortlessly converge on a target provides the distinct opportunity for accurate, efficient, and consistently reliable inputting of information. In reality, it presents a chance for the youngster to get clear and stable messages about what is being seen. The result is a significant and meaningful confidence that comes with knowing and believing in oneself. A child is now able, in a most positive way, to become the person he or she truly is.

It doesn't matter if treatment comes from perceptual, motor, and/or physiological techniques, because that only determines the methodology through which trust is developed. The question to be answered is which treatment approach or, better still, which combination of treatment approaches best serve the desired outcome. The approach that ultimately develops a global and effortless response of all systems involved in the action is the most desirable.

This much is certain: once individuals become responsible for creating change in their environment, they create the experience that comes from their own particular point of view. They become the creator of the phenomenon observed and the changes that are internalized. Accepting one's own true self results in a lifetime of enjoying one's own achievements, while at the same time recognizing and living with one's own true limitations. Knowing the difference is essential to it all.

The reservoir of vision is as full as the resource of love that comes from the heart. The extent that we see is a reflection of the love that we feel.

Chapter 2

Convergence

What Is It and Why Is It Important?

In my practice I have found convergence, perhaps more than any other visual variable, provides me with deep rich insight into my patient's own visual experience. It appears to influence my patients' ability to know themselves.

What is meant by convergence? By convergence I mean the ability to turn one's eyes inward so that each eye meets at the same common single point. Then, once convergence takes place, one can focus on that common single point in order to achieve clear and single vision. Problems quite understandably occur when one's ability to achieve convergence to a particular target of regard is deficient. One can clearly see the result of this deficiency in the character, Non, in the movie *Superman 2*. He, along with General Zod and Ursa, was able to come to Earth from Kryton for the sole purpose of ruling Earth. One of their super talents was to shoot laser beams of light from their eyes, destroying whatever the beams intersected upon. Our somewhat goofy Non could not get his beams of light together, no matter how hard he tried. His problem was his deficient ability to converge his eyes.

Recognize that, when one converges to a point in space accurately, the brain potentially can calculate depth perception or the distance an object is perceived to be from the viewer. What evolves from that is an ability to know where one is relative to an object of regard, establishing where one's body or position in space actually is. One must know one's position in space before knowing where the object is. This is considered in Kraskin's levels of commitment in the Introduction. Where objects are perceived to be is all relative to where one is in space. The term for this is called "egocentric localization/process."

So, if we consider the boy who has difficulty playing baseball, or the girl who misses continuously with jump rope, or the child with an exaggerated reading disability, is there a common cause? These problems may certainly be caused by the fact that the children's eyes are not teamed and focused properly. They do not line up at the same point or, if they do line up at the same point, that point is either in front of or behind where convergence should be taking place, at the target of regard. A common understanding of this can be related to a child who either swings a bat early or late while trying to hit a baseball. A child swinging too early sees the ball closer than it actually is: over-convergence. A child swinging late sees the ball further away than it actually is: under-convergence. Clearly, the result is a child who is visually uncoordinated and subsequently disconnected from what he or she is looking at.

I feel most vision-related learning/reading problems are associated with a lack of convergence, because I believe that convergence is one of the functions, if not the main function, for acquiring visual information. Convergence is first on the scene during visual exploration and it supports the orientation of a child's body in space to whatever it is that he or she is physically encountering. Consider convergence as the motor component of centering, where it is and, more importantly, where the child is in relationship to other objects within his or her space, again the egocentric process. Once children have located what it is that they want to inspect, say the words in the book, *See Jane Run*, through their ability to converge to the object of their regard, they can then activate their focusing ability or the accommodation system for clarity. Accommodation is the motor component of identification, what it is and what meaning can be derived from it. Convergence locates that there is something on the page and accommodation identifies what is recognizable: words on the page. One cannot identify until one can locate what it is to be identified. And, just to take it to one more level, one can't locate where it is until one has oriented to it, coming to balance with one's body and the task at hand. Again, this considers Kraskin's levels of commitment stated in the Introduction.

Consistent with this thinking is the idea that convergence is linked to one's ability to orient one's body in space.

Think of a ballet dancer going through a pirouette. As she goes through the turn, her head turns around first in order to pick up a visual anchor, a target across the room that she can line her eyes up with. Once she has locked her eyes onto the target, she can then turn the rest of her body around, staying upright because of the visual control on the anchor, holding her body upright. Or think of balancing your own body on one foot and then closing your eyes. Clearly, the greater challenge to balance will occur with eyes closed.

So now you can begin to see how convergence helps to connect and anchor ourselves in space and to the objects within that space.

In this chapter, I am trying to make clear all that convergence function is and all that I believe it can be. In so doing, I will try to make simple something that may appear paradoxically complex. I believe convergence function to be so very important that I want to try to demonstrate just how significant it is.

Convergence function helps answer the most basic questions about where we are and who we are in relationship to space and to the objects we encounter in that space. When we converge to a point in space with accuracy, our brain can determine just how far away this point in space is: our depth perception. When we know where this point in space is, we have reference to where we are in that space: our body or position in that space awareness.

Generally speaking, we know ourselves relative to where we are and what we perceive. Without an ability to view the world properly, we really cannot know— we can only infer—who we are relative to what we see based on where we see it. It follows then that when depth perception is hindered by a lack of convergence function, who we perceive ourselves to be, our identity, is hindered as well. This relationship between perception and identity provides a valuable window for one's self-understanding. How comfortable we are in relationship to our world is enhanced through our own sense of self. I believe the ease with which we experience this sense of self within our individual space world is proportional to our awareness of the difference between illusion and reality.

Al Sutton, a first generation behavioral optometrist, states that it has been said that you do not fully understand where you are or what direction you should take unless you know where you have been (2006). I believe that convergence, the ability of the two eyes to gain simultaneous information about our position in space, significantly supports our knowing where we have been. Elliot Forrest, second generation behavioral optometrist states, "It is a reasonable assumption that how an individual reacts to people, things and events reflects his attitude not only about people, things and events but, more importantly, about the self" (1984, p.3). Forest previously stated that different starting points can often lead to greatly different conclusions even when based on similar evidence (1976). In much the same way, I contend that the way in which each of us converge to an object of regard determines, to some degree, our basic beliefs and helps us to solidify our own premise. So, the question arises, how do we perceive differently as a result of having evolved with two eyes instead of one? What is the outward physiological and the inward perceptual impact or difference between having two eyes or only one?

The visual metrics of convergent function is relatively simple to measure, but simple doesn't necessarily mean unimportant. To demonstrate the impact of convergence on the internal you, I'd like you to do a little exercise with me.

I'd like you to begin by considering the world as a room. No matter where we go, our lives play out within this room, within its well-defined spatial boundary. Even when we are outdoors, we can still think of the outdoors as still being part of that room. We can easily do this because our ability to perceive, to move, to act in, as well as have an influence on, a place is always bounded by some limit; even if it's a distant horizon instead of a wall, there always exists a boundary. And we know ourselves relative to what we perceive within that boundary, as well as knowing ourselves relative to the boundaries themselves. And if something is outside the boundary, we don't perceive it and thus, for all intents and purposes, it doesn't exist for us.

Now imagine that I have presented you with a picture of a large room. This is not supposed to represent your room; instead think of it as merely a two-dimensional picture representing a three-dimensional room, any room. There is an important distinction here; note that a photograph on flat paper is almost always a 2-D analog for our 3-D world. The photographer's technique often replicates the effort of a monocular (one-eyed) viewer attempting to see the world binocular (two-eyed). Flat representations of dimensional space can therefore serve as a helpful tool.

Look at everything in this room—the picture room—as if you had just walked into it. Your brain processed a myriad of information about this place. Where am I in it? What are the boundaries in it? Where are those boundaries? How close are the objects in the room? How large are they relative to me and my location? Am I safe here? Am I in danger? Do I have room to move about freely? Do I have the autonomy to influence the objects in the room?

Sight without depth perception provides us with insights about how children with deficient convergence function answer these questions. We all see shape, we all see color, we all perceive pattern and some texture, but with compromised depth perception we lack some critical relative data that accurate convergence would otherwise provide. For example, are objects large or are they just close? Are objects small or are they just far away? Which is illusion and which is reality?

As stated earlier, without the ability to view the world through two eyes, by converging onto the objects we are viewing, we can't really know who we are relative to where we are and what we see. At best, we can only infer. If we, any of us, and that certainly includes the child struggling in school, can't accurately perceive depth or is limited in some way in the perception of space, our sense of boundary will be compromised.

Without the ability to ascertain where they are relative to the objects in their space—in their world, if you will—children can only guess at the answers to questions concerning perception of their space. And those guesses, those inferences, can certainly be inaccurate. For these children, knowing the answers about themselves are hindered by not having accurate spatial information about their location relative to spatial reality.

Beyond a doubt, efficient and accurate convergent function gives the beholder some of the answers that enable them to discover their true sense of self by knowing better how to function in their space world. And while the complex question of how vision helps to convey to children who they potentially can be still persists, I believe that one important element to understanding the answer to the question most assuredly does exist. That element relates to the comfort children have connecting to their space world as can be seen through their sense of self and through the ease with which they are able to distinguish between spatial reality and illusion. In children, developing the confidence to know *where they are* and therefore subsequently *who they are*, becomes key to knowing their true self.

Convergence function has the potential to help us all know those answers. Ralph Emerson has written, "To believe your own thought, to believe that what is true for you in your private heart is true for all men; that is genius" (2003, p.63). In my work with children, I strive for them to experience nothing less.

Chapter 3

The Difference Between Good Eyesight and Functional Vision

One afternoon a freckle-faced ten-year-old little boy sat down in my exam chair and proceeded to tell me about how he had hit two home runs in his little league baseball game. He was ecstatic because only last year all he ever did was strike out. He not only struck out in baseball, but he was striking out in school as well. His concerned parents had been told by his previous eye doctor that his eyes were fine, he had 20/20 vision. So, vision had been ruled out as the cause.

For years he and his parents had traveled from one doctor to another trying to find out why their bright young boy could not read or learn as well as his peers. As a result of his learning difficulties, he had been placed in a class for the perceptually impaired, and was receiving remedial reading and psychological counseling, all at the same time. Not only was this child not able to have playtime with the other kids, but his situation did not seem to be getting any better.

His parents became aware of behavioral optometry's vision therapy from parents who had gone through the same series of frustrating events with their own child. They too had been told that their child's eyes were fine, he had 20/20 eyesight.

The eye exam in both cases revealed that, while they each indeed had 20/20 vision, they both suffered from an eye muscle imbalance. As we have discussed, eye muscle imbalance is a condition that affects focusing and its relationship with eye coordination and tracking. It's no wonder that, without the ability to properly focus and coordinate, reading, and for that matter all other visual activities such as hitting a baseball, was indeed a difficult task: a task so difficult that no amount of remedial reading or psychological counseling could ever hope to ameliorate it.

Symptoms of eye muscle imbalance are quite varied. Some of the more common effects are blurred vision and headaches. Additionally, while reading, one or more of the following may occur: eyestrain, double vision, losing place, skipping lines, omissions, the inability to focus and concentrate, and the need to reread in order to comprehend. Youngsters with this condition very frequently read slowly and laboriously, and become easily fatigued and ultimately distracted. There are some children who simply avoid reading altogether, or, as a result of missing or substituting words, will not fully comprehend what they have read.

Eye exercises prescribed by behavioral optometrists are the treatment for these children, and yes even adults, who have reading disabilities that include one or more of the symptoms stated in this book. Vision therapy not only improves the tracking, focusing, and eye coordination skills involved in reading, but also has the potential to improve coordination in other areas such as hitting home runs in little league baseball. Keep in mind that activities outside the realm of school and formal education are not limited to sports. Children with focusing and/or eye coordination issues can similarly experience difficulty and frustration in their informal educational pursuits, such as hobbies and outside interests.

An eye exercise program for children is most effective when used in conjunction with the appropriate team of allied professionals, dependent on the child's additional needs. When this team approach is utilized, magic can often occur. I knew of such a moment when the parent of my little leaguer walked into my office and gleefully exclaimed, "Guess what, my Justin picked up a book and read, all by himself today!"

There are simply too many times that a youngster is examined by an eye doctor who states that the child's eyes are fine because he or she sees 20/20. This frequently leads a school's child study team and parents alike to falsely conclude that the child's vision is not a cause of the problem. As a result, the cause of the problem is missed and that child's problem will continue to be misaddressed. When that happens, when the symptoms are continuously treated while the cause itself is unwittingly ignored, there can be no hope of remediation. The vexing problem will continue to exist with little hope of resolution.

Children should be made aware of the joys and rewards of reading and learning. They deserve to have the benefits of knowing what their problems are and what solutions are available to remediate them.

In Psalms, it is stated, "The eye perceives only the form of something, not the substance." Vision, however, is associated with conceptual perception as one would say, "I see his point" or as scripture says, "My heart saw much wisdom and knowledge." Recognize that an eye sees form whereas vision encompasses what is perceived within.

As you continue to read, I hope you are gaining a better understanding of the importance of the totality of vision in the learning process. I hope that you are now beginning to understand that one obvious message is that a marginal eye examination is a waste of time and money when it comes to finding the root cause of a visually related reading or learning problem. The takeaway message here is that a vision problem is not necessarily because of eyesight, but rather it often results from a focusing and/or eye coordination problem. I cannot stress this enough: *bright children will often see 20/20, but they may still not be able to comprehend what they have seen.*

Vision, one of the primary elements in the learning process, if not *the* primary one, is so much more than 20/20 vision. Just about any eighth grader can tell you what 20/20 vision means, but parents and educators alike often don't know how little it means in the process of learning.

Darroll Boyd Harmon, noted physiologist instrumental in discerning the relationship of vision and body posture, discussed vision's role in human behavior. He states:

> The primary function of vision, biologically, is related to the determination of space relations and the space movements of the organism. Only secondarily, as a "higher" function of abstracting and symbolizing space movements for later facilitation and reduction of movement, is vision an "image" function, biologically. (Harmon 1958, p.14)

All that just to say that vision's primary role is to explore space and only secondarily is vision needed to extract and process what we've seen.

The following highlights strategic components of functional vision and how they can affect your child. Difficulty internalizing visual information can involve deficiency in the areas of fixation, following, focus, and fusion.

- **Fixation:** The eyes must be able to stop their movement and fixate (line up their eyes with a target they are looking at) on an object. Children who don't do this are easily distracted and usually have a short attention span. This condition may contribute to and/or be blamed on hyperactive-type behavior.

- **Following:** The eyes need to move freely in all directions: left, right, up, and down. The ability to both track and sequence information develops from this skill.

- **Focus:** The eyes must maintain a clear focus, not only on an eye chart across the room, but also on a near target. Individuals unable to do this spend additional energy simply trying to see the print in front of them. Imagine trying to read with eyes that function like a broken movie projector. Another problem people face is the need to change focus quickly. Can they see a chalkboard assignment, switch to desk work, and back again?

- **Fusion:** A person must take signals from each eye and coordinate or fuse them together to create a 3-D image. This skill is necessary for good depth perception. Does your child have an unusual fear of heights or does he or she not fear heights at times when it's appropriate? Two eyes simultaneously looking at the same place at the same time potentially tells us where the object is and where we are in relation to that object. Knowing where we are gives us a sense of who we are in that context.

Once visual information has been received, its organization and integration are dependent on perceptual skills that have developed over time. A framework of some of these essential skills include body awareness, laterality, bilaterality, directionality, form reproduction, and spatial organization.

- **Body awareness:** The ability to sense one's body mediated by nervous elements in muscles, tendons, and joints, and stimulated by body movements and tensions. The sensory experience derived from this source is called "kinesthetics." Children who have a lack of awareness of their body may experience postural and/or tonal dysfunction. They may fall excessively and/or bump into objects within their surroundings.

- **Laterality:** The ability to maintain efficient use of each side of one's body independent of the other. This ability is the prelude to crossing the midline of one's body, movement from one side of the body to the other (the beginning skill of bilateral interaction).

- **Bilaterality:** The ability to maintain efficient, integrative, and symmetrical body posture. Eye coordination and symmetrical movement are related to this skill.

- **Directionality:** The ability to recognize left from right, and up from down. A child with poor directionality is likely to reverse letters and numbers when reading and/or writing.

- **Form reproduction:** The ability to receive and reproduce form. A child must be able to recognize symbols (a, b, c, etc.) in order to make sense of them.

- **Spatial organization:** The ability to be aware of and interact with one's position and/or objects in space. Lack of this ability may result in clumsiness, disorganized motor skills, and an inability to perform puzzles. Disorganized reading and/or writing skills can result.

Identifying visual dysfunction begins the process of overcoming your child's struggle.

PART II

OVERCOMING BLOCKS AND UNLOCKING POTENTIAL

WHAT IS VISION THERAPY AND WHEN IS IT NEEDED?

Chapter 4

Vision Therapy

History and How It Works

Vision therapy or visual training is the art and science of developing, improving, and enhancing visual skills, perception, and performance. Vision therapy combines optometric training with behavior modification through biofeedback design. This combination allows individuals to become aware of their visual difficulty, control it, and ultimately reintegrate that control into effortless function. Simply put, vision therapy utilizes remedial procedures to modify and improve the way eyes and their link to the brain performs. While the therapy activities may seem simple, they are designed to correct what can be a complicated series of vision problems. Parents are delighted when their children read the eye chart with clarity, and are pleased and relieved to learn that Justin and Jaime have 20/20 vision. However, as you have already learned, that leaves the picture incomplete, for what the eye chart assesses is "sight acuity," not vision.

As we have discussed, there are two sets of eye muscles that comprise the entry point of sight into vision: one muscle system controls focus for clarity and the other controls the function of seeing single, not double. When these two muscle systems function without coordination or, rather, independently, symptoms of eyestrain and/or avoidance behaviors result. Again, some classic symptoms include eye rubbing, headaches, squinting, seeing double, closing one eye while reading or writing, missing or substituting words while reading, difficulty finishing homework, and not reading at all.

Here is a short history of the various techniques used in vision therapy programs. As you will see, the techniques used today have evolved over time. From previous entries in various professional journals, we know that as early as the 1920s, orthoptics (the ophthalmological term initially used for eye exercises) and vision therapy were based on establishing the coordinated use of two eyes and the development of the freedom within the accommodative/convergence (focus/coordination) relationship. These practices were broadened in the 1930s to include the addition of visual skills such as rotations, fixations, accommodative facility (the ability to adjust focus), and the acceptance of convex plus lenses at near point, to reduce the avoidance response. In the 1940s the motor concept of vision and skills involving peripheral fusion (awareness of periphery or side vision) were added. An understanding began to develop relating visual posture to body posture and showing how motor development could affect visual development. Further, the extension of coordinated motor systems into space helped consolidate the concept of a visual space world, and ultimately crystallized the realization that many functional aspects of vision, to a great extent, need to be developed.

My vision therapy program utilizes a series of sequenced activities and techniques designed for patients to become increasingly aware of their visual function so that remediation and alternate strategies can be elected. A program typically consists of a minimum of 48 half hour weekly sessions interspersed with re-evaluations every eight to ten visits. Therapy sessions optimally should not be longer than an hour and a quarter and should have a minimum of one day between sessions.

When problems are discovered early, before academic lags and secondary frustrations set in, the procedure is relatively simple. The longer the condition exists, the greater the opportunity for emotional and behavioral dysfunction to develop, setting the stage for the failure syndrome and for points of resistance to evolve.

Larry MacDonald, first generation behavioral optometrist, stated:

> As one examines one's own behavior, be it visual or otherwise, one is often caught in the inconsistencies in the way he has put it all together. These inconsistencies constitute resistance points and seem to limit information processing. Through awareness of the inconsistencies, one is better able to reorder the information processing system and remove obstacles that impede the development of a particular skill or integration of particular energies. (MacDonald 1972, p.1165)

Some children who receive vision therapy and who have difficulty changing an existing motor pattern, or skill, have been observed to sob or cry, may become nauseous, and can develop headaches. These collective responses have been labeled "critical empathy" and are actually an indication of progress, through subsequent positive change in visual function, within the vision therapy process. However, what may appear as a change in visual function can have a deep underlying effect on a patient's total behavior.

Bruce Wolff, first generation behavioral optometrist, was one of the first to term the expression "critical empathy" (see MacDonald 1972, p.1162). He did so when he noted that, during a vision therapy session, some patients were reported to have become uncomfortable and even tearful. Patients would initially appear unable to change a familiar motor pattern or a specific visual skill that they were earlier able to perform. In other words, they were unable to learn how to change the way in which their vision in relation to their bodies performed a particular task. Critical empathy is that challenging point, a stress point in vision therapy as discussed by Robert Pepper, first generation behavioral optometrist, (see Gottlieb 2005), when patients need to reorder or rematch their visual space, modifying existing visual habits in order to generate new integrations that no longer fit comfortably with previously learned behavior. Children, who are more adaptable and far less entrenched in their behavior, will more easily move through the critical empathy experience. It should be noted, however, that not all patients involved in vision therapy overtly experience critical empathy behavior.

Wolff (MacDonald 1972, p.1162) noted that, once critical empathy was experienced and subsequently resolved, the visual therapy that followed was of a different quality. Patients more easily generalized the ability to reorder their existing motor patterns. Thus, critical empathy constituted a breakthrough, and having been through this, patients were more capable of re-organizing their visual space and able to attain individual visual goals.

How does critical empathy relate to a child who is now in vision therapy? While some patients in vision therapy do not appear to go through the critical empathy experience; many others do. Among those who do, the experience may vary from very mild to extreme. It may be so mild that it is thought not to have taken place at all. It could also be so extreme that it involves uncontrolled sobbing, dizziness, and nausea. As I stated previously, it is true that children are less set in their ways, and so, for the vast majority, vision therapy can easily work through most challenging experiences. As with all therapy, it should be performed with support that includes large measures of understanding and love.

I include this chapter to help parents of children going through vision therapy to understand that while vision therapy frequently involves some simple changes, they are nevertheless significant changes for a child. MacDonald states, "When Optometrists are attempting to develop modification of visual behavior, they become aware that what appears to be a minor modification of visual habits may in fact have deeper underlying implications in terms of total behavior" (1972, p.1164).

Now here's the important part: most children experience some level of critical empathy. Directing them away from the activities that trigger the resistance to therapy will deter them from achieving the goals of therapy. It is my opinion, based upon over 35 years of practice with countless youngsters, that many apparently unassociated excuses for discontinuing treatment, such as conflict with another activity, length of the program, and monetary concerns often could be attributed to a child's complaints or lack of success stemming from the potential critical empathy experience. It is primarily because of that belief that I work with children the way I do. And it is because of that belief that I want every single parent of every single child in vision therapy, with me or with any other therapist, to provide that child with a loving, supportive, encouraging environment in which the experience of the therapy will be easier, and hopefully not only successful but also enjoyable.

This is how I gently guide patients through the critical empathy experience when their therapy "hits" that crucial point. I deliberately choose a particular technique that has previously elicited a critical empathy response. I then provide the patient with an age-appropriate explanation attempting to clarify the association of the difficulty of the task with the signs and symptoms that have been expressed. The severity of the expression and the stability of the patient's responses determine whether or not I advance or retreat in the treatment modality. I always exercise caution when engaging children. Understanding child development, psychology, and emotion, incorporated at each moment of the critical empathy experience, is crucial for success. When children become trusting of the process, their therapeutic experience can proceed. Psychological counseling may be warranted for some children going through a difficult critical empathy experience.

A case that exemplifies the critical empathy experience comes to mind. A young woman I had previously worked with was diagnosed with a classical convergence insufficiency (inefficient convergence) for which I began treating her. Her progress reached a plateau in just a brief period of time. I discussed with her the fact that her progress had reached a plateau for some unknown reason.

After gaining her trust, I was able to probe just a bit further with her. It was then that she confided that, each time she converged to a particular degree she would get a flashback to a traumatic event she had experienced a year earlier. When that association was made, relating her trauma with convergent posture, she was able to rationalize the fear that she had felt. She was then able to overcome her anxiety and proceed with her treatment in a more comfortable way.

Trust with my patient is most important. Cultivating a child's trust is absolutely an essential key to success.

Chapter 5

How Vision Therapy Can Aid Learning

Is it *your* child who is not visually ready for school? Well, in her cumulative record is a simple notation, "Sara is a hard worker who generally works to her capacity, it's just that she is slow in her learning." How monumentally unfortunate, that your little girl has already been labeled a slow learner—sort of code for below average intelligence—when in fact she is a very bright little girl who just isn't visually ready for the grade in which she finds herself. Unless, you, her caring parent or concerned professional, based on other clues and cues, determine that she is far brighter than her achievement level and you take action on her behalf, she may never develop into the beautiful human being for which she has the full potential to become.

It is easy to say that many bright children struggle with learning. Why? Can it be that vision, a significant contributing factor in a child's ability to learn and to respond to classroom instruction, is not held potentially responsible when education goes amiss?

Going by everything you have read so far, children who are performing below average might indeed have learning issues that are in no way related to short comings in intelligence. Their difficulties may be related not to a lack of intelligence, but rather to a dysfunction in what is simply known as visual processing.

Learning is achieved through the interrelationship of complex processes, one of which is vision. Visual information-processing problems may result in children becoming overwhelmed the very first day they enter school. The academic curriculum is designed on the assumption that children possess certain visual information-processing abilities, as well as other skills, commensurate with their chronological age. It is quite possible that the child who has not yet developed the required level of visual skill may not be visually ready for school.

Vision processing is multifaceted and complex in its relation to learning. The vision system is comprised of the eye itself, visual performance, and brain function. The eye component considers eye health, visual acuity (sight), and refractive error (eyeglass prescription). Visual performance is inclusive of eye movements (tracking), focus (accommodation), and eye teaming (binocularity). Brain function is responsible for higher levels of visual information processing, some of which are inclusive of sequential and spatial process, organization/integration, form reproduction as well as resultant visual memory. Clearly, each component of the vision process needs to be functioning at its optimum level to establish the appropriate resultant level of learning consistent with the level of development of our young.

Now you can see that there are many elements of vision that affect a child's ability to attend to and respond to a teacher's instruction. It is well known that refractive error or eyeglass problems such as nearsightedness, farsightedness, and astigmatism, all of which can result in blurred vision or eyestrain, can affect how a child performs in the classroom. However, it is also relatively common for a child to have a focusing problem that does not allow him or her to rapidly change focus from desk work to chalkboard and then back to desk work again. A child may have difficulty using both eyes together, not allowing him or her to keep words and letters single. Words may actually go into two, double, or seem to jump or move on the page. It is quite common for me to ask children if they see double. They typically respond by saying, "Yes." Their parents then ask them why they never told them. Their children quizzically answer, "Don't you see two?" It is also possible that a child may have difficulty controlling eye movements. This often results in inaccuracy, displaying common symptoms of loss of place when reading, frequent guessing of words, the need to use one's finger to maintain place while reading, or other much more subtle difficulties.

Children can elect to try to overcome visual obstacles or dysfunction by increasing their extra effort, compensating for the lack of efficiency of visual function, and subsequently interfering on a secondary level with visual information processing and ultimately with learning. Here the children are thinking about making their eyes stay on the book rather than thinking about what the words mean in the book.

Resulting difficulties may manifest themselves in a variety of ways such as, but not limited to, problems with reading, writing, mathematics, spelling, thinking, sports, and playground activities, and even social relationships involving siblings and peers. Visual deficiencies and visual information-processing defects occur in older individuals as well, supporting the fact that children do not simply outgrow these deficits. Early intervention has the potential to result in full remediation.

Treatment for learning difficulties related to visual processing consists of lenses, prisms, and vision therapy. Recognize that treatment does not directly treat learning or reading disabilities. Rather, treatment is directed to improve or, in many instances, remediate visual inaccuracy and/or inefficiency, and the resultant strain and stresses of compensatory efforts directed towards visual function and subsequently towards visual processing. Removing the visual obstacle has the potential effect of allowing your youngster to be more responsive to educational instruction.

This in no way precludes the need for other forms of treatment necessary for a multidisciplinary approach to learning. Removal of children's visual limits, however, frees them to attend to what they are looking at rather than trying to maintain their eyes on the page. It is simply shifting effort from trying to force eyes onto a page into processing the information on the page. This takes one more positive step toward the development of your child's true potential.

That potential is challenged when our children begin their academic career unprepared in their ability to process visual information. Let's look at your child entering the learning arena.

Kids entering the school arena makes me think of the seven dwarfs in *Snow White*, when they march off to work each day in single file, singing, 'Ho! Ho! Ho! It's off to work we go.' But no, it's not the diamonds we seek in caves that we mine. It's something far more precious: it's the excavating of new thoughts and ideas from within the minds of our children.

> Fall, a season of change, represents a time when our young typically go back to work digging through the caverns of their minds seeking the diamonds that represent the wealth of our future. Those diamonds represent our children reaching their individual potential. It is our children upon whom we ultimately depend on today for the betterment of life for all our tomorrows.

There exists a great need to understand what your child ultimately represents, and to support and guide that child at every age. And so we place enormous efforts into structuring our educational systems in order that children can learn with ease. We carefully and thoughtfully arrange the school curriculum so that it coincides with the appropriate stages of childhood development. We match the expectation of learning potential with the expectation of matured capability.

At age five, children start kindergarten. This is a time when vision, auditory, and kinesthetic awareness begin to become integrated. Here children learn through their work with fine and gross motor activities. By seven years of age, visual motor skills are dramatically emphasized through the reading and writing demands of second grade, matching a sense of integration between fine motor systems and speech and language skills. As a child nears junior high school, there is a sense that integrated skills have been mastered. This is the time for children to begin to acknowledge social, emotional, and physical issues, as well as worldly ones. Current events and personal health issues are presented with the hope that our children will take that major step and begin to add their own individuality to the pool of knowledge that they currently possess.

We don't stop here, simply matching development and curriculum, but go further by making sure that our children are healthy. Pediatric and dental examinations are mandated yearly. Assessment and remediation of speech and language skills are available, and occupational and physical therapy are utilized when it is deemed appropriate.

The pitfalls in education

What then goes wrong with a child who becomes, for one reason or other, incapable of climbing the ladder of success? A child who, as a result, falls into the mire of resource rooms, special education services, psychological counseling, and even the possibility of repeating a grade or two. With all that we know and with all that we do, what could possibly have gone wrong with the child who is said to be intelligent yet is having so much trouble learning? When we go back to the beginning of this process, we can see an answer to the enigmatic question, Why can't my bright child learn?

Sensory and motor skills necessary for academic success not only have to be present and normal, they must also integrate and reciprocate with each other at appropriate levels of a child's development. If one were to recognize the actions and influences of each system involved with the task of learning, the immediate pertinence of the visual system upon these actions and influences would become obvious, especially when the primary task faced by every student throughout their education is visually deciphering the printed page.

Therefore, all three sensory motor systems—vision, auditory, and kinesthetic—involved with integrated information processing needs to be matched with overall development. The educational curriculum must be in tune with the perceptual processing of each system. Here we have the circumstance where auditory and kinesthetic processing have become reconciled, yet vision, the function through which upwards of 80 percent of information is processed, is left out.

Why do we leave vision out of mandatory yearly evaluation? Think about it: upwards of 80 percent of a child's information year after year in grade after grade is processed through vision, yet, astoundingly, child study teams evaluate a child, perhaps your son or daughter, without consistent input and concern about his or her visual welfare.

The situation becomes further clouded by the mainstream reaction to commonly asked questions concerning vision. Most often a child suspected of having difficulties in visual processing will come back from their eye exam with a report of, "Eyes okay, this child has 20/20 vision."

These children see eye doctors who do not recognize the implications of visual processing deficits. Herein lies a major stumbling block. Educational systems may not recognize that vision is an entity that can be redeveloped or modified in a way that significantly affects the learning process. These eye doctors themselves erroneously believe that 20/20 vision means "Eyes okay." Then add to that number the well-meaning members of the child study team who are confident that vision is not involved in the child's learning difficulties because of their lack of knowledge about what vision truly entails. How many times is it heard by the child study team, "We can eliminate vision as a cause of her problems," and yes, you guessed it, "The eye doctor reports that she has perfect 20/20 vision."

The question that needs to be addressed if we are to make significant changes in the learning capability of our young is clear. How do we educate professionals, who affect the education of our children, about behavioral optometrists and their care for children with functional vision disorders, and about how these disorders are associated with learning? Even more important, how do we eliminate the false understanding of professionals in education with the idea that vision can't affect learning and that it can't be redeveloped?

A solution that would answer these questions and more is mandatory early and annual visual evaluations by eye doctors who will assess and treat visual-processing disorders. In addition, these same eye doctors need to be integrated within child study teams in order to direct programs aimed toward remediation of visual dysfunction. The truth is vision as a process can be changed, and inappropriately adapted visual behavior can be modified to improve visual function. This improvement is crucial to the educational well-being of our children. Only with cooperation among disciplines will there be an understanding of what children need. In order to ultimately reach the greatest potential within an educational/learning system, vision as the primary sense must be preserved. The greater the preservation of vision and its integration with sensory motor systems, the more children will experience and enjoy greater success in learning.

Dyslexia

One major consequence in misunderstanding the visual process is the inappropriate use of the term "dyslexia." At the start I want to clarify that, when I use the term "dyslexia" in this regard, I use it in reference to dyslexia as it is commonly associated with reading inaccuracy and/or instability, not true developmental dyslexia. True developmental dyslexia which will be further addressed in the book, is characterized by severe difficulties in recognizing and decoding letters or words. I am using the term here because many children unwittingly diagnosed with dyslexia, in reality, may simply have some form of visual dysfunction discussed in this book. Therefore, I'd like you, the reader, to begin to associate common usage of the term with visual dysfunction. A behavioral vision assessment can determine the difference.

'Dyslexia' is a word, however, that reminds me of a Superman comic book villain called Mr. Mxyzptlk. He was a small man from another world who would make a nuisance of himself here on Earth. The only way our man of steel could rid our planet of this pesky intruder was to fool him into saying his name backwards, "kel-tip-zix-um," which would return him to his home in the fifth dimension. Immediately Mr. Mxyzptlk would vanish, leaving his words behind saying, 'I will return.'

Even though we'd all like our children to go away at times, they are very much with us after they reverse what they have seen or read. What is not so funny is that some of these children, on their own, sort of vanish. Oh they don't vanish from sight, but they do withdraw into themselves: so much so that they might as well have gone to a different world. Their frustration, of not being able to read and write like all the other kids, can begin to take its toll. It can make children feel as if they are worthless. And that is a powerfully negative feeling. It is so powerful and so negative that some of these children do vanish into another world, a world of their own deep within. It is a world separate from their parents and from their friends. But unlike Mr. Mxyzptlk, many of these children return from their own dyslexic world when they are at last able to read and write in a correct and accurate manner.

The first step in correcting this problem comes with the recognition that there is a problem, and that there is a sound treatment for that problem. This is the most difficult step a parent can take, but, once initiated, the problem emerges from one that is insurmountable to one that has a stable and specific course of treatment with the results that parents are looking for. Because of the possible multiple nature of the condition, a team of educational professionals certainly may be necessary. In other words, whenever appropriate, the school's child study team should be involved.

Many dyslexic children have a number of problems at one time, but the two most common are in the areas of vision and/or language delays. Visual problems related to dyslexia are usually obvious and easy to diagnose and treat. Symptoms often include reversals, loss of place and skipping of lines while reading, reading words that are not on the page, omissions, double vision, and sometimes avoidance of reading. The child who avoids reading may not be lazy at all, but simply frustrated at not being able to read as well as his or her peers.

A behavioral optometric vision therapy program specifically tailored for each child is the treatment of choice for these children who have reading disabilities that include one or more of the symptoms described throughout this book. Eye exercises are often used in conjunction with the appropriate special education team. When the team approach is used, magic often can and does occur. I have witnessed this throughout my career.

Only with the conclusion that a visual problem is not solely dependent upon a child's eyesight but, rather, also dependent on tracking, focusing and/or eye coordination problems, will our children re-emerge. So long as anyone associated with treatment for children who are struggling in reading and learning do not understand this premise and the reasons why, those children stand a good chance of not having their needs met. This failure to address the visual needs of our children will not be because of a lack of good intentions but because of a lack of knowledge about vision.

All children with reading problems must have their visual systems fully evaluated. This means that they should receive a vision evaluation far beyond the simple determination of seeing 20/20 in order that they may experience the joys and rewards of reading for a lifetime.

Remember, Mr. Mxyzptlk was able to come back from time to time. Well, unlike Mr. Mxyzptlk, children diagnosed as dyslexic, who are not tested for eye muscle imbalance or focusing problems, can be lost in their own world of jumbled letters and words forever.

Chapter 6

Vision Therapy and Learning Disabilities

A significant segment of our children are not being successfully educated by our current mainstream educational programs. This is true even though serious well-intentioned attempts have been made by boards of education to bolster educational systems with therapeutic services. Nevertheless, the success at individualized education remains unimpressive when your child is the one not able to learn. As stated throughout this book, the lack of success is due, in part, to a lack of exploration into the role that vision has on reading and learning.

Children experiencing learning difficulties have been given various labels: developmental alexia, developmental aphasia, minimal neurological dysfunction and maturational lag, minimal brain dysfunction, and, more recently, attention deficit disorder (ADD).

Developmental dyslexia, although represented by a small segment of the pediatric population, estimated to affect between 5.3 percent and 11.8 percent of school-aged children, may be additionally included and defined as a severe inability to learn or read through deciphering symbols. Despite adequate intelligence, and education, difficulties may include word decoding and recognition, spelling, and subsequent reading comprehension (Taub

2011). Directionality skills are often underdeveloped, resulting in severe reversal of letters and words. Recognize, though, that mild reversals are part of normal development, typically reducing through the third grade. Academically, the true diagnosis of developmental dyslexia suggests a diagnosis of exclusion. What this means is that, if there are any physical conditions that could create the symptoms presented, those physical conditions must be corrected before developmental dyslexia can be diagnosed.

On the other hand, forms of reading disability are prevalent in as much as 20 percent of school-age children. That's one in every five schoolchildren. I'd say, without fear of contradiction, that that represents a problem seriously in need of a solution.

Reading disorders are a prominent and ever-present concern that is a subset of learning disabilities. And they may be accompanied by other academic disorders in varying degrees. Then there are the children who fail to learn to read or even fail to learn in general in spite of average or better than average intelligence, average or better than average motivation, and average or better than average educational opportunity. These children have experienced normal auditory and kinesthetic development, normal acculturation, have no evident brain damage, and experience no primary emotional disorder.

Nationally, the estimated prevalence of children with a learning disability ranges from 4 percent to 15 percent, with most teachers estimating that 4 out of a classroom of 25 children had, have, or will experience learning problems. If one considers a conservative estimate of the total school population in the US of 46 million children, then the number of children with some sort of learning disability ranges from 1.8 to 6.9 million.

Recognize that this is not a homogenous group, but rather one that crosses lines of color, religion, social class, and national origin. Clearly, one may assess that an epidemic of learning disabilities truly exists within the US.

Although children with learning and reading disabilities are often active, they are not always hyperactive. They are, however, often distractible. They exhibit a short attention span and can be characterized as impulsive. This leads a child toward premature closure, allowing little time between thought and execution. The ultimate effect is to cut down on the amount of information being processed at any one moment in time. Extraneous and irrelevant head, eye, and hand movement further confound the issue.

Subgroups within learning disability

There appears to be two apparent subgroups in learning disabled children. Those completely free of associated social, emotional, physical, and economic factors, and those who are not. The latter group is significantly greater in number. Each group requires a significantly different treatment approach based on the associations made.

Research has clearly associated prenatal, perinatal, and postnatal disorders with subsequent disabilities. Prematurity, low birth weight, forceps deliveries and trauma experienced at birth have been implicated. Delays in gross motor skills such as movement through space, buttoning, lacing, or cutting are cause for concern in children during the first half of first grade. These activities are established with visual and/or tactile feedback that guides the motor response.

Delayed speech and articulation correlate as well with learning and reading delay, which often result in subsequent language disorder. A delay in vocabulary and syntactic development during the primary grades is typically indicative of an innate language handicap.

Although little support has been shown for mixed dominance as a cause of learning disabilities, ill-defined laterality has been found to be of greater significance. This can lead toward difficulties in left–right discrimination and a component of a child's lack of lateral awareness in conjunction with a poor sense of directionality in space.

Nutrition has been implicated in this learning and reading disadvantaged milieu. One needs to recognize the significance of socio-economic disadvantage with regard to nutritional deficit in order to understand its relevance.

The complex of attention deficit hyperactivity disorder (ADHD) represents a distinct group of children who are distractible, inattentive, and hyperactive with an underlying impulse theme. Although they have a significant representation in the learning disabled population, they may in fact represent a specific subgroup whose treatment needs to be specialized.

In addition to not being able to perform academically, the learning disabled child begins to learn how not to perform emotionally. I have stated that these children begin to feel that they are what's wrong, rather than understanding that they are limited in some specific way which can be corrected. These are not just school disabilities, they are life disabilities. These emotional reactions can include defiance, withdrawal, acting out, regression or even aggression.

Misunderstanding vision roles

Often economic pressure coinciding with a misunderstanding of how learning disabilities develop stands in the way of appropriate treatment for these children. In particular, in 1981 the American Academy of Ophthalmology and, as recently as 1998, the American Academy of Pediatrics in concert with the Committee on Children with Disabilities, the American Academy of Ophthalmology, and the American Association for Pediatric Ophthalmology and Strabismus denied the relationship of visual dysfunction, in the areas of eye tracking, focus, and coordination, to learning disabilities as outlined in this book. As a result, we see special education programs that continue to address symptoms and not causes.

The American Academy of Optometry, the American Optometric Association and the College of Optometrists in Vision Development have responded with *Vision, Learning and Dyslexia: A Joint Organizational Policy Statement.* They state:

> Learning is accomplished through complex and interrelated processes, one of which is vision. Determining the relationships between vision and learning involves more than evaluating eye health and visual acuity (clarity of sight). Problems in identifying and treating people with learning-related vision problems arise when such a limited definition of vision is employed. (1997, p.98)

A multidisciplinary approach, one that combines the skills of a variety of professionals, is in order if we are to effectively reach those in need of special services. The dysfunctional trail extends from the physical/ physiological to the perceptual and, ultimately, to the emotional. This is why it takes an evolved and enlightened team approach to truly meet the needs of children with learning disabilities. This begs the question, Does vision have a rightful place in our child study teams?

Only with cooperation between disciplines will there be more of an understanding of what children need. In order to ultimately reach the greatest potential within an educational learning system, vision as the primary sense must be accepted. The greater the preservation of vision and its integration with other sensory systems, the more children will accurately experience their world and, as a result, enjoy greater success in learning.

If your child is struggling in school and not attaining success, it is necessary for you to find out the workings of the referral process in his or her school. When you become more directly involved with the education of your child—that does not mean interfering, it means involvement—your child will benefit.

Identifying learning disability

So, your struggling youngster is simply having some sort of a learning problem, a learning disability. By its very words, a learning disability means that a child is having difficulty learning caused by some sort of limitation. Although children with learning disabilities may be bright, for some reason they have difficulty learning with the ease that their intelligence would suggest. It is not all that unusual to find an intellectually gifted student with a learning disability. As you might suspect, children with learning disabilities usually have difficulty keeping up with other students at their grade level. And it is not necessarily about a lack of ability; instead, it is often because of some impediment to their learning process. Such children tend to work harder to keep up with their peers. Motor skills related to performance such as writing, copying, or even sitting in a chair for age-appropriate periods of time produce stress. These children often complain about their eyes or simply avoid using their eyes. Additionally, it is not at all unusual that they also complain about neck pain and pains in their hands, as well as their trunk, when they are asked to sit for prolonged periods of time. Frequently, teachers describe such students in any one or more of the following ways: lazy, fidgety, agitated, sloppy, tense, or even anxious. Hopefully, such a child will be identified as one with a possible learning disability. When this happens, as mentioned earlier, the identified child will almost always be referred to the school's child study team.

Likely outcomes of referral

There are three possible outcomes for the child referred to the child study team. The first outcome is that the team properly identifies the cause of the problem and that the child receives the best possible help that the particular school and/or school system is able to provide. When it comes to the child, your child, most particularly if he or she suffers from an impediment to their learning, effort doesn't count: only results do.

The second possible outcome is that the child is diagnosed as learning disabled and yet, as I point out earlier in this book, that child may receive treatment that merely addresses his or her symptoms and not the root cause of the problem. Thus, for the most part, the problem continues and the parents, the members of the child study team, and, most importantly, the child continue to experience frustration. That frustration can negatively impact the child sometimes, unfortunately, irrevocably.

The third possible outcome is that the child study team deems the child as not in need of special services. Again, nothing in this book is intended to demean child study teams. When viewed in their entirety, the accomplishments of the US education system are indeed outstanding. But that is not to say that some learning disabled children don't fall through the cracks; some do. Sometimes the fault lies with the financial abilities—or should I say inabilities—of a school district to afford the additional specialists needed to identify some rather difficult to identify causes of learning disability. At times there are other causes, but with the same result: a child who is in need of services continues throughout education without those services.

It is always necessary that you, as a parent of a child with a learning disability, do everything that's reasonable and practical to be certain that your learning disabled child receives all the services to which he or she is entitled. When the school agrees to have your child evaluated by the child study team, be certain that a behavioral optometrist is either on the team or that an examination by a behavioral optometrist is included as a part of the evaluation.

In a case similar to the boy previously described who hit two home runs, a mother who had been referred to me by the mother of one of my other patients described her daughter as being exceptionally bright, yet having all sorts of learning problems in school.

Examination of this girl revealed that both her right and left eye functioned at 20/20. I then proceeded to check the ability of both eyes operating at the same time. Herein lay the problem: the muscles controlling focus of the left eye were more inefficient than those of the right eye. Because eye focusing and eye coordination are linked, the fact that one eye focused with a muscle that was more strained than the other eye, resulted in the two eyes not being able to work together efficiently.

This girl had what to her was normal vision—after all, it was what she had experienced all of her life—blurred vision whenever she changed focus from one distance to another. It was no wonder she was having difficulties in school. The more she focused on making her eyes work, the less she was able to concentrate on what she was looking at, trying to process or understand what the words she was looking at meant.

Further, testing revealed that the mother's assessment was correct: this was indeed an exceptionally bright girl and another case of a parent knowing—just knowing—that something was wrong and that that something was not her child. Through vision therapy and an appropriate therapeutic eyeglass prescription, the condition was ameliorated. Although she still needed the resources of remedial reading to help bring her up to the level of her classmates, she no longer had the burden of her visual dysfunction. She now had the appropriate skills needed to learn and read efficiently.

What is so very disturbing is that parents generally know when something is "just wrong"—or "just not right"—even though there may be little recognition of the problem by others. Parents in such instances are merely told that they are expecting too much or simply that their child is not trying or not capable. Now, and this is very important, when you as the parent feel that something is "just wrong" or "just not right," it is your responsibility to pursue the answers you seek no matter what other professionals may say. You know when you are "just right." Children with learning disabilities will benefit from you joining in their struggle.

Chapter 7

The Role of the Behavioral Optometrist in the Child Study Team

So, your daughter is still having difficulty in school. You know that she is bright. You know that she can do the work. It just isn't happening, despite the fact that you have provided an atmosphere conducive to learning in your home. Yet, she is still not learning. She rebels at the prospects of long assignments. Gee, lately she even rebels at the prospects of doing any homework at all. She is interested in a wide variety of subjects, yet seems to have no interest in reading about them. In desperation you turn to her school's child study team.

A child study team typically consists of a chairperson, the school psychologist, a social worker, the learning and/or reading disabilities teacher or consultant, an occupational and physical therapist, and speech pathologist. A referral may also be made to a pediatric neurologist. These individuals, acting in good faith and within their range of expertise, gather information that they have been trained to gather, that the law requires them to gather, and that experience has led them to believe is important to gather. Nothing here is in any way intended to question their competence. As previously stated, and worth repeating, is the charge to the schools of America: "Educate all the children of all the people." If you take just a moment to think about that charge, then you will agree that with all its faults the system of education in the US is indeed remarkable, and, while easily criticized, actually needs to be commended.

Let's take a closer look at the makeup of a typical child study team. A child referred to a school's child study team for possible classification and help is given a well-thought-out workup.

The school psychologist conducts a comprehensive battery of evaluations intended to assess the intellectual, social, and emotional development of the child.

The social worker conducts a case study to evaluate factors within the family or community that may be contributing to the student's learning difficulties. He or she will usually look into other factors that have the potential to serve as support resources.

The learning and/or reading disabilities teacher or consultant conducts an educational assessment. It is this child study team member who does an evaluation of the nature and potential causes of the learning and/ or reading disability confronting the child. He or she determines the child's educational strengths as well as weaknesses, and looks for areas in need of improvement on a functional level. At times, the diagnosis of dyslexia is questioned. Again, know that this diagnosis is a diagnosis of exclusion. Any physical correlate, auditory and/or visual manifestation of the condition must be considered first before the diagnosis of dyslexia can be made.

The occupational therapist evaluates and treats sensory and motor integration delays in a child ranging from gross to fine motor development. He or she will work with basic issues of coordination as well as handwriting concerns. Physical therapists will often work with issues surrounding muscle tone and motor development. Treatment will concern itself with increasing muscle strength, flexibility, and balance.

The speech pathologist assesses and establishes therapeutic treatment for receptive and/or expressive difficulties in speech.

The pediatric neurologist considers physical and/or medical conditions contributing to a child's difficulties. They consider the possible diagnosis of ADD or ADHD, which often follows with a recommendation of medicinal treatment such as Ritalin. Similar to the diagnosis of dyslexia, physicians should initially consider all physical reasons that may be contributing to a child's difficulties, before resorting to medication. In other words, they should be obligated to consider all functions that could duplicate the symptoms that the child is experiencing. Auditory, sensory motor, environmental, emotional, psychological, and of course vision are some considerations that, if found to be dysfunctional, must be considered and treated before medication is given. If medication is utilized, but a misdiagnosis exists, multiple attempts at prescribing different medications and dosages will not have significant effect. A child may appear to act out less and have improved focus, yet the inability to learn still threatens. The misdiagnosis may undermine the situation further because children can learn to believe, even more deeply, that there is something very wrong within them, and that the medication is simply covering it up with an additional layer of distraction. Recognize that the symptoms of ADD and ADHD are very similar to those of visual dysfunction. The major difference is that ADD and ADHD are typically experienced in two or more separate environmental settings—for example, school and home—whereas visual dysfunction is task specific. In other words, the symptoms are most prevalent when involved with visually demanding situations such as reading and writing. If these steps are taken but to no avail and medication is found to be appropriate, its effect will be quick and quite successful in treating ADD and ADHD.

The chairperson, along with the members of the team, meets with the parent, in this case you, or the guardian of the child, and together, based upon all the collected data, work up an individualized educational plan (IEP) for your daughter. And, oh yes, don't forget, an eye exam may have been called for as part of the information-gathering process. And let's not forget either that a superficial eye exam may have yielded the result: 20/20 vision in both eyes.

> The following is what I can only call a tragedy. You sit in on this meeting convinced that all avenues have been explored. The school has even paid to have your daughter's sight evaluated. You, basking in your limited knowledge of vision, sit at the meeting just as convinced as all the members of the child study team, in their limited knowledge of vision, that vision has nothing to do with the child's learning problem. How sad, when in reality eyesight may not be the cause of the problem: but vision may.
>
> You are led to the false conclusion that sight is not the cause of the problem. As I have mentioned in numerous chapters, 20/20 vision in both eyes is hardly enough if both eyes are not working together.

Remember the analogy of 20/20 vision as a house. If vision as a process is represented as a house, the role that 20/20 plays can be considered to be the door of the house. Clearly, the door is important in order to enter a house or the eye in this case, but it is only that part of the house or eye that allows the information to enter. The remaining house is the entirety of vision itself.

And so the child study team, armed with all the information at hand, labels your daughter a slow learner or some other negative label, gets her prescribed medication, and decides on an IEP to give her the help she supposedly needs. Unfortunately, if misdiagnosis exists, the plan is designed to treat the symptoms. So long as your daughter is receiving extra services from the school, you may go on falsely feeling that you are doing all that you can for her. And, yes, the members of the child study team and her very well-intentioned teachers feel good that they are doing all in their power to help her as well. In the meantime, the root cause may remain.

Now I am not saying that all learning and/or reading problems are caused by eyes improperly working together, what I am saying is that the ability of two eyes to properly function together is an essential factor in a child's ability to read and ultimately learn. The visual component in a child's learning and/or reading difficulties must never be overlooked because, if it is the cause of the problem, treating symptoms will never solve the riddle or complete the puzzle.

I urge all parents, educators, and health professionals to insist that a comprehensive behavioral visual examination be given, at the least, to all students who struggle in school.

> Your daughter may not be in need of special classes or a special program. Use your power to advocate for what she does need.
>
> I want the same thing for her that you do: I want to see her eyes light up with joy as you hand her the next Harry Potter book to read.

Chapter 8

Vision Therapy and Occupational Therapy

A Co-joined Approach

Let's see, your child seems bright enough yet is still experiencing some difficulties in school. That raises an interesting question, a question that, while perhaps interesting to me, is far more perplexing to you—namely, Is your child perceptually impaired, and are you, the parent, in need of discovering how *your* child learns? This indeed is a most important question. In this context, perception relates to the ability to organize and integrate sensory motor stimuli as opposed to abstract concepts.

The symptoms of perceptually impaired children are as varied as the individual personalities they present. How then do we go about the process of knowing which children are not developing and learning successfully as a consequence of their perceptual skills? Children who do not have trouble perceiving what they see sail through a multitude of experiences building self-confidence. Those who have difficulty, however, stick out in the crowd. You can find them waving a red flag. And the message on that flag is so very clear, "I am stuck."

Perceptually impaired children are often identified as being immature. A characteristic of such children will be their difficulty in sitting and playing. Inattention, impulsivity, and distractibility become hallmarks of their behavior. From this immature behavior comes what we all dread as parents, the unsuccessful child. Lack of success begins with an inability to learn and all too quickly develops into academic failure. There may first be an aversion to learning colors, letters, and even tying shoes or buttoning buttons. Once children begin to internalize feelings of frustration, the problem shifts from one of learning to one of self-confidence.

No one seems to have all the explanations for such a complex problem. Yet there are some explanations if we begin to look from a different perspective. To begin with, our children's perceptual problems stem in part from our inability to understand their learning process. Not all people learn in the same way, and, most assuredly, your child may not learn in the same way you do or, and this is most important, in the way his or her teacher does.

Still another part of the problem is the way in which our educational system functions. There may be an inability to correlate information from specialists in related disciplines specifically trained in the area of perceptual development. In fairness, schools most certainly attempt to correlate information. They do so within a child study team approach. These teams individualize the education of our youth by identifying strengths and weaknesses and developing programs accordingly. In spite of all these laudable efforts to develop specialized programs, many of our children still fail to thrive academically and/or socially and remain at risk. They simply fall through the cracks.

Behavioral optometrists view a perceptual problem from a different perspective than those in education or in medicine. That difference is in the understanding that, when visual perceptual demands exceed a child's ability to perform, lags in development will occur, causing delay in processing vision and, ultimately, a delay in learning. This is important because even though some children may appear to perform adequately in school, they still may not be performing to their potential. Parents will often say to me, "My child just doesn't work to his potential." Once intellect, or your child's ability to adapt, is outweighed by his or her demands to perform, learning delays will become obvious.

When we speak of vision process or any process for that matter, we are speaking about the interrelationship of three components comprised of input, organization/integration, and output.

Consider the analogy of a computer, which incorporates a keyboarder, keyboarding information (input), and software organized for a particular program (organization/integration) needed for some particular purpose (output). Behavior acts in a similar pattern.

Individuals receive information that then directs their perception to organize and integrate past with present in order to develop ideas or concepts on the subject. If we break down these concepts into finer components, we end up with a sensory motor integration model of processing. The component parts of this model look something like the following.

Internalization-Organization-Storage-Retrieval-Utilization-Behavior

- **Internalization** represents inputting of information from three principal sensory and motor systems comprised of (1) kinesthetic or body knowledge, (2) speech and language through auditory function and (3) vision. There are four components inputting visual information; eye coordination/convergence, focus, eye movements, and refractive error or eyeglass prescription.

- **Organization/integration** represents body awareness, laterality, bilaterality, directionality, and spatial organization.

- **Storage** represents short-term memory.

- **Retrieval** represents an ability to search for and to bring out information.

- **Utilization** represents an ability to use information retrieved.

- **Behavior** is the resultant reaction to what was received.

My approach in treating perceptual delay considers the importance of internalization—that is, input skills. It is these skills that set the tone for other components to develop within the visual process. It has been shown that improvement in input skills alone has had positive effect on the development of the other skills that follow in the process. In other words, improved input will support and develop improved organization/integration, short-term memory, retrieval, and utilization, and ultimately can result in behavior that represents a positive sense of self, a self-confidence. That's not to say that perceptual therapy in organization/integration will not have a positive effect, but I do believe that the practical effect of treating and remediating input first is dramatic. I believe it has the ability to completely remediate certain presentations of visual dysfunction.

The following case highlights the clinical relationship between input and perceptual skills.

A 6-year-old child was referred to the office for an evaluation for perceptual delay by his first grade school teacher. The teacher felt that he was not working to his ability and lately was becoming disruptive in class. He had trouble sitting in his seat, would jump off his seat, speak out at anytime and often trip and fall. Writing and copying were quite laborious, he was unsure with right and left concepts, and he had a tremendously difficult time sustaining any length of desk top tasks. It was becoming impossible to keep his attention during group story time. Upon evaluation, utilizing a comprehensive eye exam and vision therapy workup, I did find delay in all of his perceptual skills as well as inaccuracy in his eye movements and inefficiency in focus and eye coordination. Recognize, I said inefficiency in focus and eye coordination. As in most situations, eye muscles are stronger than they need to be. What is inefficient is the message that the brain sends to the eye muscles. Think of a radio dial turned slightly off the station. That static message is what is being addressed in a therapeutic program. Once the brain can send the appropriate clear message to the muscles it desires, visual function is on the road toward remediation.

There was no significant refractive error; the child did see 20/20 but did not read the eye chart crisply.

Rather, he hesitantly had to spend an inordinate amount of time trying to discern the letters.

I prescribed a therapeutic progressive bifocal (one without the line across the lens) of mild strength, and a prism for constant wear. Vision therapy was prescribed as well as a referral for an occupational therapy evaluation. If the presenting symptoms were simply about visually sustaining desk top demands, a referral to the occupational therapist would not have been made. However, in this case, although I thought that improvement in the perceptual area would result from improved input, I didn't feel it would be enough to remediate and I did feel that this child's visual and perceptual difficulties could be remediated.

Treatment was initiated in both vision and sensory motor skills through the visual therapy and occupational therapy programs. The vision therapy focused on input skills while the occupational therapy primarily centered on the sensory motor. Again, in this case I felt the sensory motor difficulties were significant enough to warrant co-joint therapy. Needless to say, this child made dramatic and quick change in all areas of concern. Immediately, upon wearing his glasses, his teacher noticed him to be more focused during story time. She felt that his attention had improved, enabling him to focus during class presentations and desk top activities. The occupational therapist also responded in the same way, stating that he was more attentive to her tasks as well. This child with obvious and disruptive behavior became one of the top-performing children in the class, and not just this class but all his other classes to come. He went from a depressed little boy to one who always had a smile.

Behavioral optometry's use of lenses, prisms, and vision therapy is specifically designed to correct your child's eye muscle imbalance and the associated perceptual delay that may result. Behavioral optometrists, who see perception from a different point of view, are sorely under-utilized in the search to improve the perceptual development of our children.

Bobby, a 9-year-old boy, can further illustrate behavioral optometry's relationship with occupational therapy.

Bobby had been referred to an occupational therapist by a learning center. Bobby was thought to be above average in his academic ability by his parents even though his academic achievement did not support this view. This was another case where the parent "just knew" that something was wrong even though no one else seemed to agree.

The occupational therapist evaluated this boy over two sessions. Bobby's mother's concerns were based upon Bobby having become increasingly agitated at home, including a resistance to doing homework, and his considerable discomfort when he was expected to produce written work.

Bobby's tests indicated that he had normal muscle tone and a normal range of motion that was more than adequate to support classroom performance. Below normal scores were indicated in tasks requiring bilateral integration such as jumping jacks. His ability to hold postures was deficient for his age. Additionally, he was unable to perform other tasks involving rhythmic movement. He seemed to be experiencing a number of physical inefficiencies that were interfering with his ability to perform in the classroom setting. He displayed an immaturity in the integration of the two sides of his body, an immaturity of function that was interfering with age-appropriate movement patterns. Even though he tested in the normal range, his fine motor skills demonstrated a lack of control. Attention difficulties appeared to underlie a number of sensory and motor weaknesses, and to contribute to poor use of visual and motor abilities. Most interesting to me was that, when motor output was removed from perceptual testing, his scores were in the above-average range. The occupational therapist noted symptoms of visual discomfort throughout her testing of Bobby. These included his head moving close to the page while reading and writing, a head tilt with body rotation, and eye pain. She suspected visual problems. Her suspicions were enhanced because Bobby was able to perform certain tasks with greater alacrity with his eyes closed; then he was dramatically more relaxed, and showed marked improvement in motor fluency.

The occupational therapist referred Bobby for a visual assessment. Now it was my turn to see if I could confirm the visual elements of his impediment to learning. In short order, I discovered that he had poor tracking skills. He had a tendency to lose his ability to follow (track) a penlight target. During my assessment of his tracking ability, I noted that his left eye occasionally jumped ahead of the target. Additionally, I noted a midline jump; that is, his eyes had difficulty moving smoothly from one side of his body to the other side without jumping when he got to his midline (the middle of his body). This represented a potential delay in motor development. Bobby also presented with spasm of his focus while turning his eyes inward (convergence). His eyes appeared to get stuck. I thought that an explanation for his eyes getting stuck at his near point of convergence (the closest point in which he could keep both eyes together while turning inward) was possibly due to his over-focused visual system. That most often occurs when an individual is over-adapting or compensating for an underlying binocular inefficiency. As I moved the fixation point closer, Bobby had difficulty letting go at near point. It became necessary for him to blink in order to let go.

I noted that he had to move within three inches of the paper when asked to complete tasks that involved writing. At one point he turned his body completely sideways simply to draw a diagonal line. Additionally, I noted that he tilted toward his left as he attempted tasks that required fine motor skills. He complained of pain in his left eye after about 20 minutes of eye-hand coordination activities. And, during interactions with others, he demonstrated an avoidance of eye contact. Independently, each eye tested at 20/20 and there was no refractive error noted.

Bobby met with the occupational therapist once a week for 9 months. His progress with her was immediate and most impressive. Throughout this period, he also continued treatment in vision therapy, attending 48 therapy sessions. I experienced similar remarkable gains in his ability to perform. At the end of 9 months, he achieved grades of almost all As in the highest level math and reading classes. His handwriting became far less effortful and his written work showed marked improvement. Happily, his mother found that he was able to finish his homework in a reasonable amount of time and without disruption to the family. His excessive anger and resistance were gone.

The occupational therapist and I believed that the simultaneous, co-joined intervention of occupational therapy and vision therapy facilitated the significant improvement Bobby experienced. He is now a happy boy functioning without the conflicts at home caused by his limitations. He is experiencing a high level of success in school more commensurate with his high level of intelligence.

This case, as we discussed earlier, particularly demonstrated that sometimes the parent "just knows" and that co-joined therapy is remarkably effective.

PART III

SPECIFIC VISION PROBLEMS AND BEHAVIORAL OPTOMETRIC INTERVENTIONS

Chapter 9

Types of Lenses and How They Help

The question, often faced by teachers and parents alike, is why some children who are intelligent lack the ability to easily learn to read or, subsequently, read to learn. How to properly address the problem facing these "slow learners" and "slow readers" is one that continues to plague educators.

It is commonly understood that the act of reading is essentially a process whereby the reader matches visual signs with existing speech-auditory organization. Children who have difficulty reading to learn, yet present with the ability to use words and sentences to express themselves appropriately, indicate the potential cause of the reading difficulty to be more of a visual than an auditory problem.

Speech development readily takes place as young children experience their world, connecting significance to what is being seen. Along with this, children also encounter the cultural demands that are associated with the printed page, demands that have the potential to create difficulty in matching visual configurations with a more advanced speech-auditory system.

The complexity of the reading act is one that involves the total organism. It is known that growing children tend to move away from environmental stresses that get in the way of natural development. This is especially true of those activities that tend to demand a more focused concentration. Consequently, near visually centered tasks bring on what is for children a predictable avoidance response. It is a response based upon their involuntary nervous system. In other words, children who laboriously and without profit engage in the act of reading have an inherent drive to escape from the task. Their choice is to physically move away from the task, cease from the thought process of the task, or distort themselves through adaptation in order to somehow succeed in the task. In Chapter 10, we will discuss how some children who are academically successful develop progressive degrees of nearsightedness throughout their school years as a result of their adaptive response to succeed.

The analogy that comes to mind in seeking an answer to the question concerning children who experience reading as a laborious activity relates, strangely enough, to monkeys. When a monkey grooms its mate, it will do so diligently for a few seconds, and then look up and away for three times the length of that diligent grooming period. Certainly, having children stare out the window for three minutes for every minute they read is not the answer to the question. Children need to create a congenial visual environment within which reading and the ultimate learning process can and, even more importantly, will occur. For this to happen, it is essential to match visual and speech-auditory experiences while at the same time addressing, and hopefully satisfying, the avoidance response.

Lenses

A spherical convex spectacle lens has properties that both allow an individual to visually process within a near-centered visual task and also address the avoidance response.

> Think of the time when you held a magnifying glass up to the sun and directed the focused light in order to burn a hole in a dry leaf. The distance of the focused light to the magnifying glass was based upon the power created by the curved or rounded exterior of the magnifying glass (convex lens).

A convex or learning lens in spectacles allows children to focus their eyes with less effort, by the lens doing part of the work. This enables children to maintain focus on near-centered visual tasks, such as reading and writing, with less effort and without the need of an avoidance response.

A bifocal lens provides the means for a learning lens to be positioned so that the bottom part of the lens is available for near visual tasks while the top part of the lens is positioned for visual tasks at distance. The far point, or distance lens, is positioned on the top part of the lens while the bottom portion contains the near point learning lens. If distance vision is not compromised, there is no need for the far point lens to contain any lens prescription at all. When that is true, the clear distance lens is provided to prevent far distance blur that would be experienced if one were to view a distant object through the near point learning lens at the bottom. Simply put, a bifocal allows opportunity for all academically related tasks to be performed in a classroom without the need to remove the eyeglasses, and of course, with less effort.

Recognize, however, that these glasses do not correct "eye problems." Rather, these lenses protect against developing "eye problems" or "ocular defects." I use lenses most often, full time, in the classroom for all visual demanding tasks and vocational purposes. However, some prescriptions may be removed for sports and other physical activities depending on the child's needs.

Lenses prescribed for classroom and vocational use for children who experience learning difficulties not only make near and far tasks accomplishable with less effort but also have the potential to eliminate the avoidance response.

Prism lenses

Throughout this book I have tried to write primarily for parents of children with vision deficiencies hoping at the same time that other readers, such as, but not limited to, teachers and child study team members, will be able to easily understand the material presented. In as much as I often prescribe prism lenses, I would very much like you to understand why. My concern here is that it is not easy to write an easy read chapter on prism lenses. So, bear with me as I attempt to make this an "easy read" chapter.

Amiel Francke, first generation behavioral optometrist, has stated, "Lenses are an optometrist's most valuable tool" (1988, p.73). They have the ability to achieve an alteration of human behavior by changing the direction of light entering the eye.

Although prism lenses look like normal lenses in a spectacle prescription, the effect they have is quite different. They are lenses that change the direction of light rather than condense or expand light as conventional lenses do. Think of a prism as a triangular glass, bending light that passes through it similar to the way light is broken into different color wavelengths. The bottom, flat part of the prism is called the base while the top is called the apex. Light entering the prism leaves the prism bent toward the base. Now here is the significant point: when one views light that is bent in a particular direction, one's body posture can elect to make an associated adjustment to that bent light. Therefore, these lenses are typically used to enhance one's ability to rematch eye coordination in relation to coordination of one's body posture.

The term "yoked prism" was originally and presently used to differentiate it from the typically prescribed lateral prism. Yoked prisms are defined as a pair of prism lenses of equal power with their prism base in the same direction. These prism lenses are highly selective and specific. Low powers, ranging from 0.25 to 5 prism diopters (a unit value of prism lens power) are typically prescribed for in and/or out of office treatment. The direction of base is determined by the desired change in body posture while the degree of power is based on a clinician's professional judgment. In the final analysis, the true value of a yoked prism is in its influence on balance and orientation. Most often, the behavioral effect is represented by a demonstrable improvement in spatial awareness and orientation of one's body.

Children who typically indicate a need for yoked prisms clinically present with reduced awareness of their body in space related to a lack of focus, inattention, distractibility, hyperactivity, impulsivity, limited eye contact, excessive visual search, and/or perseverating mannerism. The manifesting conditions may include autism and pervasive developmental delay, asperger's syndrome, ADD, and hyperactivity, and can frequently involve as common a diagnosis as oculomotor dysfunction (eye movement disorder). The theme of a prism lens correction is that it addresses visual disorders that can significantly contribute to adaptive visual and behavioral skews which are related to the movement of one's body in space and posture.

A "vertical yoked prism" correction

A "vertical yoked prism" correction affects our ability to function in three ways.

1. Its initial effect is to raise or lower eye gaze. I most often prescribe a vertical yoked prism in the base-up position, which serves to lower eye gaze. This promotes the ability to converge (turn inward) one's eyes. The nature of our eyes is that, upon shifting into down gaze, eyes turn inward. In the same sense, up gaze promotes divergence (turn outward). Eye motor skills will initially begin to stabilize with base-up vertical yoked prism correction because of its effect on improving the stability of convergent posture.

2. The secondary effect of yoked prisms promotes more accurate convergence to a target of regard. As we discussed in Chapter 2, enhanced convergence stabilizes one's ability to know where an object is in space relative to oneself (egocentric process). One's ability to judge body movement in space will be enhanced, giving one greater awareness of one's own position in space.

3. Ultimately, postural control and balance will develop from a counterbalance shift in the center of gravity of the body as a result of an eye motor shift in gaze. It is well known by professionals educated in the field of body dynamics that, as eye gaze shifts, the center of gravity of the body, located at the level of the navel, shifts opposite to the eye movement. Therefore, a shift in eye gaze downward results in a counterbalance shift in the center of gravity of the body in an upward manner. The effect is as if one is moving backwards on the heels of the feet, creating a correction of one's body posture. A righting effect of one's body will occur, often resulting in children becoming less over-active in their behavior.

A "yoked prism prescription"

"Yoked prism prescription" represents a beginning platform upon which children can learn to rebuild a stable and efficient visual world. Now here's the point: once convergence is stabilized, a child's ability to know where an object is in space in relation to self is improved, thus enhancing spatial judgment. Ultimately, the child begins to develop better posture and demonstrates less over-active behavior.

Here is a typical clinical situation representative of a child in need of a yoked prism prescription.

I worked with a two-and-a-half-year-old little girl, referred by a physical therapist who had felt that she had gone as far as she could with her. The child was inappropriately fearful about walking down a flight of stairs and all but panicked when people, or things, quickly moved toward her. She presented with tracking inaccuracy, a lack of ability to sustain focus, and an unstable convergent system. I prescribed 1 unit of vertical prism, base in the upward position, and a +0.25 unit of a focusing correction to support or substitute for her focusing ability; in effect redirecting/redistributing her efforts to focus and converge. She was instructed to wear her eye glasses full time for one month. Her mother felt that she would never keep the glasses on because she was so active and inattentive. Robert Kraskin has said, "A lens does nothing to a person, but a person can do much with a lens" (2003, p.53). My response to the mother was that, if her child appreciated the benefits of feeling greater connectedness to her surroundings through the lens, not only would she wear the glasses but she would forget they were on and ask to put them on in the morning. Through the utilization of these prism/focusing lenses, dramatic progress was made. When the little girl returned after one month of wearing the prescription, her mother said that she would often forget that her glasses were on her face and typically would fall asleep without taking them off. Her negative symptoms were dramatically reduced. It was through the use of these lenses that her awareness of her body posture changed and she was able to gain accurate judgment relative to the position of her body and her surroundings. She could walk down a flight of stairs with ease and showed no fear of people or objects approaching her.

More than just life altering, her improvement was life changing. This shy, clumsy, and inhibited child was now becoming better equipped to explore and appreciate her world. She became sure about herself and happy in her new-found ability to investigate within her environment.

Chapter 10

Some Specific Vision Problems

Nearsightedness, Strabismus, and Amblyopia

Nearsightedness

Did you know that myopia, or nearsightedness, or, as the British call it, shortsightedness, is a vision problem experienced by about one-third of the population? Just what is this vision problem all about? Well, it occurs when vision for near objects is clear and far objects are blurred. Thus, as the term would suggest, objects that are near can be easily seen; a person who is nearsighted has clear near vision.

All this is common knowledge. However, what is not commonly known is that some children with this condition will not need to wear glasses at all while some are told that they need to have their prescriptions increased every few months, resulting in thicker and thicker lenses. Children who have frequent increases in their lenses are often diagnosed with functional nearsightedness (myopia) by behavioral optometrists. Typically, functional myopia begins as early as five to seven years of age and usually starts with only a slight lens prescription. Not surprisingly, it may initially be a condition commonly associated with eyestrain. It is not at all uncommon for such children to experience difficulty when copying from the chalkboard. The first symptom that usually occurs is reduced transient distance vision immediately after sustained near vision tasks. The blurred distance vision remains and gradually worsens with time and the overall demand of the near visually centered task.

Functional myopia is different from genetic myopia in that genetic myopia is passed on from one generation to the next. This happens regardless of how the genetic recipients use their eyes. The genetic form of nearsightedness typically starts earlier, generally between two and five years of age. It begins with an initial prescription of moderate to even high lens power, and is typically not associated with the eyestrain experienced with near visual tasks.

Eyestrain, which ultimately translates into nearsightedness, begins with excessive use of the internal eye muscle (ciliary muscle), which controls the focus of the eye. Focusing strain may occur as a secondary result of an adaptive process initiated by a lack of coordination—or inefficient coordination—between the six external muscles (extraocular muscles) that surround each eye and the singular internal muscle controlling focus. These six muscles of each eye control the turning inward of the two eyes. That is, 12 muscles in all need to coordinate in order to turn the eyes inward together. Lack of coordination of these external muscles may cause the internal focusing system to over-compensate, causing an eye muscle spasm. This potentially occurs because the internal and external muscle systems are linked, allowing one system to support and compensate for the other. Typically, extra effort to focus is needed when there is a lack of ability to coordinate and turn the two eyes inward. Even though nearsighted vision problems resulting from eye muscle imbalance are not the same as those resulting from inherited genetic myopia, situations can occur when both functional and genetic nearsightedness are present at the same time. A behavioral optometric assessment can identify and discern the difference and subsequently direct treatment accordingly.

Here is the important element in treatment. Treatment for functional nearsightedness is not the same as treatment for genetic nearsightedness. Treatment for genetic myopia is typically through the use of a nearsighted spectacle lens, compensating for the distance clarity problem. Treatment for the underlying cause of functional nearsightedness is through remediation of the eye muscle imbalance as a consequence of vision therapy and a therapeutic lens prescription.

Treatment for functional myopia may include a therapeutic eyeglass lens sometimes in the form of a bifocal, prism lenses, vision therapy, proper visual hygiene, and a diet designed to reduce stress and strain of the visual system. The eyeglass lenses are designed to reduce the need to over-focus by substituting with a focusing lens. The prism component of the lens further reduces focusing strain through its support of convergence, taking away the need to compensate with over-focus. Vision therapy has the potential to integrate skills eliminating the need to compensate one system for another. Proper vision hygiene may include diffused uniform lighting and proper posture. In addition, some recent research suggests that a properly balanced diet rich in chromium may actually reduce myopic effects. A nutritionist should be consulted for best results.

There is still a lot that is not known about nearsightedness and its development. However, there are proven programs and procedures that may reduce and/or eliminate nearsightedness for your child today. If your son or daughter is exhibiting symptoms that may indicate functional myopia, head for the nearest behavioral optometrist as soon as possible. The sooner a child receives treatment, the more effective the result and the greater the chance that functional myopia will not develop.

Strabismus

Strabismus is a condition that affects approximately 48 out of every 1000 children. It not only affects cosmetic appearance and limits function, but it also creates havoc with the ability to trust what is seen, and, thus, how children ultimately feel about themselves. How sad but true it is that so many of the visual limitations children experience have an adverse impact on their own self-image, and strabismus is one of them.

Strabismus includes three major conditions: esotropia, exotropia, and hypertropia. Esotropia refers to the condition where one eye turns inward toward the nose. This is commonly referred to as "crossed eyes." Exotropia refers to eyes that turn away from the nose. The common term for this is "wall eyes." As one eye tends to turn outward more than the other, it often appears that the person is not making direct eye contact. Less common is the condition whereby one eye actually points higher than the other. This condition is called hypertropia and often results from birth trauma, eye muscle surgery, and/or serious head injury. An even less common condition is called cyclotropia. Here, one eye actually rotates around differently in each eye or turns about the axis, or center of the eye, differently in each eye. In all of these conditions the eyes do not, in fact cannot, work together.

Strabismus is the broader term used to mean one eye is pointing in a different direction from the other. Symptoms of this condition may include double vision, suppression (the turning off of one eye in favor of the other, or one eye turning off the ability to process information), gravitational insecurity (the inability to have confidence in knowing position, or body in space related to objects in an immediate environment), words jumping, words moving while reading, reading words that are not on the page, distortion of depth perception, and confusion. Some children have an extreme fear of heights while others lack any fear at all, both causing concern. As you can readily understand, all these symptoms are potentially great impairments to learning. Most unfortunately, treating the symptoms and not addressing the underlying effects can lead to frustration and negative feelings about self. Addressing the ultimate ability of the two eyes to work together in harmony begins to address the frustrations and lack of awareness of self.

The onset of strabismus can occur at different stages of development. However, the greatest frequency of eye turning is within the first year of life and between the ages of two and five years.

It is a common event for children under the age of six months to have fleeting times when their eyes don't appear to be working together. Most times these are normal situations when coordination skills are in the process of being developed. It is also common for an infant to turn both eyes inward at the same time as they learn to explore and experience the spatial world closest to them. As long as their eyes do not remain inward over significant periods of time, the experience is normal.

What is of great concern is the situation where the two eyes stay uncoordinated. When there is an infrequent length of time that the two eyes are working together, a lack of experience of depth perception develops. Researchers have reason to believe, through their work with cats, that, if the two eyes are not working together by two years of age, there is little to no chance that depth perception will ever be realized. The reason for this is that binocular, or two-eyed cells, in the cortex of the brain are believed to have a critical period of two years during which the development of these cells occur. Research has suggested that after two years of age binocular cell development ceases. Therefore, it is most important that parents of infants with an intermittent or constant eye turn have a consultation well before the two-year period is up. Recognize, however, that the research is not absolute.

If the turning of the eye is constant, or even frequent, patching the eye that is not turning is often utilized as part of the therapy program. Children should be engaged in visual activities while being patched. This enables the turned eye to have the opportunity to improve sensitivity and ultimate function. Patching regimens also include time when both eyes are given the opportunity to coordinate simultaneously. When this form of therapy does not yield the desired result, surgical intervention by a pediatric ophthalmologist may be considered. If surgery is decided upon and when the eyes are consequently physically aligned, vision therapy can fine-tune visual function, supporting efforts to maximize the two eyes' ability to work together. Note that eyes pointing straight as a result of surgery doesn't necessarily mean that they function together.

From the ages of two to five years there is significant growth and development within the visual system. Focusing and coordination become critical for exploration through localizing and identifying objects within the environment. A breakdown in the relationship of focus and coordination skills may result, at this time, leading to the development of strabismus. Excess focusing may cause an eye to cross, while inefficient or ineffective focusing may lead to a wandering eye condition. Treatment for this type of strabismus has been found to be the most effective when eyeglass prescription and therapy have begun soon after the eye begins to turn. If left alone, the extent and duration that the eye turns can increase and the adaptations of the condition become more pronounced and difficult to treat.

Once established, strabismus represents a state of confusion within the brain. Confusion, or a state of disarray, occurs when one eye tells the brain something quite different from what the other eye is telling it. Questioning which eye's information will be accepted not only delays visual response, but also tends to cause one to mistrust what is being seen: confusion. The paradox is that with a strabismic condition the greater the ability for the two eyes to function together, the more potential confusion exists. When one eye is constantly turned, one of the eyes is always turned off, or suppressed; thus there will be no conflict between messages, no confusion. Understandably, with one eye turned off, there is no rivalry of messages sent to the brain. However, with constancy of the eye turn, there will also be less possible awareness of depth perception and less of an awareness of one's body in space. This results from depth perception being limited. Recognize that, as the ability to coordinate the two eyes increases, so does the probability of increased depth perception and subsequent awareness of body or position in space, and a reduction in visual confusion.

Amblyopia

Functional amblyopia, or lazy eye, is the most common cause of monocular, one-eyed visual impairment in children. One might initially think of lazy eyes in terms of the dictionary definition of lazy, you know, disliking activity or exertion, sluggish, slothful. Can it possibly be that eyes have a preference to work or to not work?

As you may have suspected all along, the term "lazy eye" has nothing to do with the popular idea of laziness. Instead it refers to a condition caused by an active process of the better eye inhibiting, or suppressing, the poorer eye. This ultimately causes a reduction in sight clarity, or visual acuity, for the eye being inhibited. Be aware that lazy eye, or amblyopia, in this chapter, refers to a condition in which there is no pathological inhibition causing the condition. Although there are pathological reasons for amblyopia, they will not be addressed in this book. Typically, the earlier in life an eye is suppressed, the poorer the visual acuity will be.

There are two conditions that account for functional amblyopia or lazy eye. One is called strabismus, discussed earlier, which is the condition where the two eyes do not point at the same place at the same time, and the other is a significant difference in the eyeglass prescription between the two eyes, called anisometropia. In anisometropia, the eye with the higher prescription typically demonstrates reduced visual acuity. Remember, we are talking about a dominant eye inhibiting the lazy eye with no pathology involved. We are not looking at an involved surgical procedure to resolve this condition. Instead, we are looking at the proper eyeglass prescription, patching, and vision therapy to bring about the desired result.

Let's explore further. The best way to treat a lazy eye condition is to prevent its occurrence in the first place. Amblyopia screenings have been positively used by nursery schools and elementary schools to test visual acuity in young children. Those children with potentially reduced vision have been referred for evaluation and treatment as appropriate. Treatment might consist of a proper eyeglass prescription, and/or amblyopia therapy. Amblyopia therapy often includes patching regimens while engaged in visually demanding activities. The purpose of treatment would be to establish the opportunity, through biofeedback situations, for the two eyes to work together while stimulating the lazy eye to experience what it has missed. Research has shown dramatic improvement in visual acuity and resultant binocular coordination with the appropriate treatment intervention.

Mild cases of reduced vision tend to need less patching time, approximately two hours, while significant vision loss may need upwards of six hours of patching time per day. In order for gains to be maintained in visual acuity, sustained improvement in binocular skills must be established. The more improved the binocular skills, the less one eye will dominate or inhibit the other. Clearly, the more equal the skills between the two eyes are, the better the improvement in visual acuity will be maintained.

Although eye care professionals have made great strides in the treatment of lazy eye, unfortunately a significant number of children are still affected by this condition. Improvements in the screening process as well as the comprehensive way in which we treat this condition can reduce the number of children and ultimately adults affected. Parents, please note that infants should have their eyes examined within the first year of life in order to prevent or reduce the amblyopic condition. Be assured that age-appropriate therapies are readily available for infants.

The available knowledge and understanding of this condition needs to be disseminated throughout our schools and communities so that the appropriate and available treatments can be utilized to their fullest potential. The quicker the amblyopic condition is treated, the sooner the resolution and the better the prognosis. Lazy eyes that remain lazy are eyes that are uninformed.

When I Was 12

Let's go back for a brief moment to when I was 12 years old and lacking in self-confidence. I share this incident not necessarily as an event of which I am proud, but rather as one of the moments in my life that helped shape me into the person I ultimately became. Earlier in this book, I briefly mentioned that part of my life.

The detail that I didn't mention was that there was a bully in the neighborhood who had me virtually petrified with fear. He had repeatedly threatened to beat me up—a task that in my mind wouldn't take a great deal of effort on his part. I was short, I was somewhat chubby, and I was certainly insecure in my own abilities and even, as I recall, in my own self-worth.

I asked my brother the question, "What could this bully possibly do to me?" Well, the answer was that he could, and undoubtedly would, beat me up and I'd probably get a little bit bloody. Now, even at his young age my brother had some sage advice. It was the fear of the beating, he suggested, that had me concerned, not what the actual beating would be like. If, he suggested, I got the potential beating over with, then the fear of anticipation would be forever removed and my life as a somewhat normal—albeit, fat and short—kid could continue.

So, mustering up all my emotional strength, I went to the bully's house, rang the bell, and when he answered

I suggested that if he wanted to beat me up now was the time to do it. I'll never forget the look of delight that came on his face as he eagerly put on his coat and stepped outside to proceed with his dirty deed.

Now even at 12 I knew it wasn't right to deliberately hurt someone. I knew even more so that it was reprehensible (even though that word itself may not as yet have been a part of my vocabulary) to take delight in deliberately hurting somebody. Yet, that was exactly what this bully was about to do—or should I say attempt to do. I say that because, as it turned out, he ran into a slight problem. The problem was my righteous indignation (although I may not have mastered that concept yet either). Nevertheless, I became so angry at the thought of this big bully about to take delight in hurting me that, with what I am now certain was a rush of adrenalin, I actually beat the living daylights out of him. I sent him back into his house with unanticipated results– actually by both of us—bruises and a bloody nose for him and a new sense of self-worth for me.

That was a lesson that has influenced me ever since. I could, I learned, control my own destiny. The choices I make are my own. I must never let others, or the fear of failing, be a part of what I do. And, perhaps most importantly, whenever I treat a youngster, I think of that 12-year-old boy and what he had to face and overcome. As a result, I do my best to help my young patients confront their visual concerns and fears and work fearlessly to overcome them.

I invite you to join me in the ultimate resolution of your child's visual dysfunction and in the progression towards his or her true awareness of self-attainment, the self-worth such children deserve.

A Sample Letter

Over the years I have received countless letters from the parents of my young patients, as well as from the young patients themselves. Here is an example of one of those letters.

Dear Dr. Warshowsky,

As I watch my daughter happily walk onto the school bus each day, it has been on my mind often to tell you how much you changed her life and ours.

Before I brought her to your office several years ago for an examination, she was a frightened little girl. She was clumsy, afraid to move around (even in her own familiar home), and fearful of many things and strangers as well. I have never experienced this before with any of our other children. She was receiving therapy from an early intervention agency and was certainly making strides, but still withdrawn. Both my husband and I were still concerned.

When you diagnosed her and gave her a prescription for glasses you changed her life and ours! Now we have our daughter! She soon was running around the house and up and down stairs. She became involved in the activities of the house and enjoyed playing outdoors. You cannot imagine the pleasure we all had in watching her on the swings and in the playground. A pair of glasses made the world a safe place for our daughter.

I want to really thank you for helping my daughter and my family. May G-D bestow on you and your dear family only good health, happiness and success in all your endeavors.

Very sincerely yours,

(Signed by the child's mother)

Whether it's a young boy or girl who requires some rather extensive therapy or a child just requiring an eyeglass prescription, they all need and deserve what that little girl in the sample letter needed. A parent may request counsel on what direction they should take for their child. Co-joined treatment with other professionals maybe essential for optimal success. Whenever anyone seeks my help, I picture that 12-year-old little boy I once was, ever so clearly. And so, rest assured that I will be there in full and total measure.

Visual Function Self-test

Yes	No	(please tick)
		Do you ever experience double vision?
		Do objects appear to be moving when they are not?
		Are you unable to see depth?
		Do you get lost easily?
		Is it an effort to maintain your concentration?
		Do you tend to skip words or lines of print?
		Do you omit or need to reread?
		Do you feel clumsy?
		Do you bump into things as you move about?
		Do your eyes itch, burn, or water?
		Do your eyes pull or ache?

		Do you avoid sports, especially those with high speed objects?
		Do words appear to float or move while you read?
		Do you tend to spill liquids more than other substances?
		Is there a delay in refocusing when you look away after sustained close work?
		Do your eyes feel tired at the end of the day?
		Do you sometimes have to squint, cover or close an eye when looking at objects?
		Does going to school or busy places cause you to feel anxious?
		Are you exceptionally sensitive to sunlight or glare?
		Do you feel like you have tunnel vision at times, in spite of many things to look at?
		Do you have trouble navigating places such as school or large spaces?

If you have answered "Yes" to any of these questions, you should be assessed by a behavioral optometrist.

Exercises That May be Done at Home

What follows are a series of exercises designed to enhance visual efficiency. They may be easily done at home with the supervision of a behavioral optometrist, if prescribed.

1. Flashlight tag

What you need:

- Eye patch
- Poster board
- Symbols (letters/pictures)
- Flashlight

What it trains:

This teaches the eye to line up with objects of regard.

What you do:

1. Place different symbols on a poster board.

2. Place the patch on the child's left eye first.

3. Ask the child to shine his or her flashlight onto named objects on the poster board.

4. Have the child locate objects on the poster board in a random manner.

5. Place the patch on the child's right eye and repeat.

Alternative: Ask the child to shine a light flashlight onto objects in his or her environment if not able to do the above.

2. Red-green TV trainer

What you need:

- Red and green glasses

- Red plastic sheet

- Green plastic sheet

- Video/TV or computer

What it trains:

This teaches the eyes to "stay on" and not turn off (i.e., anti-suppression) dynamically.

What you do:

1. Tape the red and green plastic sheets onto the TV screen with the red on the top, green on the bottom, not overlapped.

2. Have the child put the red and green glasses on, over his or her regularly worn glasses with the red lens covering the right eye.

3. Have the child sit about three to four feet from the TV set.

4. If the child can see the whole picture (i.e., through the red and green plastic), then both eyes are "working."

5. Have the child move back one foot. If he or she can still see the whole picture, suggest moving back another foot.

If half of the screen turns black, then one of the child's eyes is suppressing. The color screen which turns black, indicates the eye that is suppressing. If the red screen is black, the eye behind the red lens is suppressing and, if the green screen is black, the eye behind the green lens is suppressing.

Have the child think about turning "on" the eye that went "off," or blink. If this does not work, have the child move a little closer to the TV screen.

Have the child watch TV in this manner for about 15 to 20 minutes, working to keep both eyes "on" and being able to see the whole picture.

Alternative: Have the youngster play a computer program with the red and green sheets and the red and green glasses.

3. Pointer in straw

What you need:

- A drinking straw and a pointer such as a pick-up stick

What it trains:

This helps to train the two eyes to work together at near point (depth perception).

What you do:

1. Have the child hold the pointer.

2. Sit directly in front of the child and hold the straw horizontally at the child's eye level with the openings of the straw to the right and left of the child's face.

3. If the child is using his or her right hand, use your right hand. Switch hands halfway through the exercise.

4. Have the child line up the pointer with the straw. Then have the child put the pointer cleanly into the straw.

To make it harder:

1. Have the child hold the pointer one to three seconds before putting it into the straw.

2. Move the straw closer and closer to the child. Stop if the child feels discomfort or sees double.

3. Move the straw a little higher or off to the side.

4. Hold the straw at different orientations: vertical, horizontal, or diagonal.

Note: At no time throughout this exercise should the opening of the straw face the child.

4. Red and green flashlight tag

What you need:

- Flashlight with a red lens

- Flashlight with a green lens

- Red and green glasses

What it trains:

This teaches the eyes to remain "on" and not turn off (i.e., anti-suppression) and to work together.

What you do:

Cat and mouse

1. Place the red and green glasses on the child, over his or her regularly worn glasses with the red covering the right eye and the green covering the left.

2. Hold one of the flashlights while the child holds the other.

3. Direct the light from your flashlight onto a wall.

4. Ask the child to then direct the light from his or her flashlight so that that light is on top of yours.

5. Continue moving your light to different places, while the child continues to move his or her light to yours.

Following

The youngster directs his or her light onto your light and continuously follows it as you move it about the room. If the child can only see one color, he or she is suppressing the other color. Should that happen, have the child think about turning "on" the eye that went "off" or have him or her blink.

5. Near/far chart

What you need:

- Letter, picture, or symbol charts, one large, one small (letter size should be determined by your optometrist)

- Eye patch

What it trains:

This teaches changing focus between far and near while keeping symbols clear.

What you do:

1. Put the eye patch on the child.

2. Hold the small chart 13 to 16 inches away from the child.

3. Hold the large chart about 10 feet away from the child.

4. Have the child read the first letter (or picture or symbol) from the large chart and then the next letter (or picture or symbol) from the small chart.

5. Repeat this until the child reaches the end of the charts.

To make it harder:

1. Have the child read the first two letters (or pictures or symbols) from the large chart and then the next two from the small chart. Repeat this until the end of the charts.

2. Have the child read the first three letters (or pictures or symbols) from the large chart and then the first three letters (or pictures or symbols) from the small chart. Repeat until the end of the charts.

3. Have the child read the first letter (or picture or symbol) from the large chart and then the last letter (or picture or symbol) from the small chart. Repeat until the end of the charts.

6. Brock string

What you need:

- Three-foot long piece of string

- Two different colored beads

- Wall hook

What it trains:

This teaches the ability to accurately coordinate both eyes together, from a point farther out in space to a point closer and then back out to far.

What you do:

1. Place the two beads on the string and attach one end of the string to the wall slightly below the child's eye level.

2. Have the child stand straight up holding the other end of the string to his or her nose while keeping the string taut.

3. Place one bead at the far end of the string and the other about one foot from the child's nose.

4. Ask the child to look at the farthest bead and describe what he or she sees. It should be two strings meeting at the far bead forming a "V" shape. The child should see two near beads and two strings that are the same height when looking from side to side.

5. When looking at the near bead, the child should see two strings meeting at the near bead and two strings moving away from the near bead forming an "X." He or she should see two far beads and the strings should be the same height.

6. If the child only sees one string, ask him or her to blink rapidly or vibrate the string with the aim of getting to see two.

7. Start moving the near bead closer to the child's eyes but to a point where he or she can still maintain one of them.

8. Alternate looking at the beads to a beat.

7. Walking rail/balance beam

What you need:

- Balance beam (1" × 5" × 8" or 1" × 6" × 8"; 2.54 × 12.70 × 20.32 cm or 2.54 × 15.24 × 20.32 cm) of common pine, sanded to avoid splinters. Traction grip tape may be applied to the beam to help performance.

- Eye patch

- Fixation charts (letters, pictures, or symbols)

What it trains:

This improves body balance, eye-foot coordination, eye fixation, and movement control.

What you do:

1. In bare or stocking feet, have the youngster walk the beam forward heel to toe, first looking at his or her feet, then fixing his or her eyes on the chart.

2. Repeat going backwards, heel to toe, first looking at the feet and then at the fixation target.

3. Have the child call out loud, in sequence, the letters, pictures, or symbols on the fixation chart going from left to right, then right to left and top to bottom as he or she is "walking" the beam.

4. A metronome can be used to vary speeds or beats, taking each step with a beat.

The beam may be raised off the floor an inch or two by using small blocks of wood. This increases the difficulty level of the exercise. Alternatively, a bean bag or paper cup can be balanced on top of the child's head and/or questions may be asked and answered in order to increase the demand level of this exercise.

If You Have Questions

If you have any questions about your child's vision, please feel free to call me at my Ringwood, N. J. office at +1 (973) 962 4488 or at my Roslyn, N. Y. office at +1 (516) 869 8717 or at the State University of New York, College of Optometry +1 (212) 938 4029 where I serve as an associate clinical professor. I can also be reached through my website: www.drjoelwarshowsky.com.

Joel H. Warshowsky, OD, FAAO, FCOVD.

Bibliography

American Academy of Optometry, American Optometric Association, College of Optometrists in Vision Development (1997) *Vision, Learning and Dyslexia: A Joint Organizational Policy Statement.* American Academy of Optometry, American Optometric Association, College of Optometrists in Vision Development, February 25.

American Academy of Pediatrics (1998) *Learning Disabilities, Dyslexia, and Vision: A Subject Review.* Committee on Children With Disabilities, American Academy of Pediatrics (AAP) and American Academy of Ophthalmology (AAO), American Association for Pediatric Ophtghalmology and Strabismus (AAPOS). *Pediatrics 102*, 5, 1217–1219.

Beck, R.W. (2003) "A Randomized Trial of Patching Regimens for Treatment of Moderate Amblyopia in Children." *The Pediatric Eye Disease Investigator Group. Arch ophthalmology 121*, May, 603–610.

Beck, R.W. (2005) "A Randomized Clinical Trial of Treatments for Convergence Insufficiency in Children." *Arch Ophthalmology 123*, January, 14–28.

Bradshaw, J. (1988) *Healing the Shame that Binds You.* Arlington, VA: Health Communications, Inc.

Bradshaw, J. (1996) *Family Secrets.* New York, NY: Bantam Press.

Emerson, R.W. (2003) "Nature and Other Writings." *Self Reliance 63,* Shambhala: Boston, MA.

Flavell, J. (1996) "Piaget's Legacy." *Psychological Science 7,* 4, 200–203.

Flax, N., Mozlin, R., and Solan, H. (1981) "Discrediting the Basis of the AAO Policy." Guest Editorial, Learning Disabilities, Dyslexia, and Vision. American Academy of Ophthalmology Policy Statement: Learning Disabilities, Dyslexia and Vision. Approved by: Board of Directors, A.A.P.O.S., 5/7/81, and Board of Directors, A.A.O., 6/27/81.

Forest, E. (1976) "Clinical Manifestations of Visual Information Processing, Part1." *Journal of the American Optometric Association 47*, 1, 73–80.

Forrest, E. (1984) "The Tyranny of the Premise: Aspects of a Psycho-behavioral Philosophy of Visual Function." *Journal of Optometric Vision Development 15*, 4, 3–9.

Francke, A.W. (1988) "Introduction to Optometric Visual Training-Training Lenses." *Optometric Extension Program, Curriculum 11, 61*, 3, 73.

Gesell, A., Ilg, F.L. and Bullis, G.E. assisted by Ilg, V. and Getman, G.N. (1970) *Vision: Its Development in Infant and Child.* Darien, CT: Hafner Publishing Company. Original publication 1949.

Getman, G.N. (1993) *How to Develop Your Child's Intelligence.* Santa Ana, CA: Optometric Extension Program.

Gottlieb, R. (2005) "Attention and Memory Training: Stress-Point Learning on the Trampoline." Optometric Extension Program. OEPF Inc. Publishing.

Groffman, S. (1978) "Psychological Aspects of Strabismus and Amblyopia – a Review of the Literature." *Journal of the American Optometric Association 44*, 9, 995–999.

Harmon, D.B. (1958) *Notes on Dynamic Theory of Vision: A Study and Discussion Outline*, 3rd edition. Dallas, TX: Harmon Publishing.

Harnden, R.J. (1990) "The Language of Models: The understanding and communication of model with particular reference to Stafford Beer's cybernetic model of organization structure." *Systemic Practice and Action Research 3*, 3, 289–302.

Kalb, L. and Warshowsky, J.H. (1991) "Occupational Therapy and Optometry: Principles of Diagnosis and Collaborative Treatment of Learning Disabilities in Children." *Journal of Occupational Therapy Practice 3*, 1, 77–87.

Kephardt, N. (1971) *The Slow Learner in the Classroom.* Columbus, OH: Charles E. Merrill.

Kraskin, R.A. (2003) "Lens Power in Action." *Optometric Extension Program Foundation, Inc.*

Levine, M. (1987) *Developmental Variation and Learning Disorders.* Cambridge, MA: Educators Publishing Service.

Luria, A.R. (1973) *The Working Brain: An Introduction to Neuropsychology.* London: Penguin Books.

MacDonald, L.W. (1972) "Implications of Critical Empathy, Primal Scream and Identity Crisis in Optometric Visual Therapy." *Journal of the American Optometric Association 43*, 11.

Piaget, J. (1969) *Development and Learning*. Ithaca, NY: Cornell University Press.

Piaget, J. and Inhelder, B. (1966) *The Psychology of the Child*. New York, NY: Basic Books.

Richards, R. (1984) *Visual Skills Appraisal, Appraisal of Visual Performance, and Coordinated Classroom Activities*. Novato, CA: Academic Therapy Publications.

Shasry, B.S. (2007) "Developmental Dyslexia: An update." *Journal of Human Genetics 52*, 2, 104–1099. Rochester, MI: Department of Biological Science, Oakland University.

Skeffington, A.M. (1931) *Differential Diagnosis in Ocular Examination*. Chicago, IL: A.J. Cox Publishers.

Skeffington, A.M. (2006) *Visions*, Newsletter of the College of Optometrists in Vision Development, Our Optometric Heritage, 6, 6, 6.

Suchoff, I.B. (1975) *Visual-Spatial Development in the Child: An Optometric Theoretical and Clinical Approach*. New York, NY: State University of New York Print Shop and Graphic Arts Department.

Sutton, A. (2006) *Visions*, Newsletter of the College of Optometrists in Vision Development, Our Optometric Heritage, 36, 4, 6.

Taub M.B. (2011) "Review of the Literature: Dyslexia." *Journal of Behavioral Optometry 22*, 2 48–49.

Vail, P. (1987) *Smart Kids with School Problems*. New York, NY: Dutton.

Warshowsky, J.H. (1994) "Optometric Vision Therapy/Training for Esotropic Strabismus Using the Cheiroscope as a Measure of Success." *Practical Optometry 5*, 6, 264–269.

Warshowsky, J.H. (1995) "Psychovisual Therapy: A Biopsychosocial Approach." *Journal of Optometric Vision Development 26*, 4, 219–223.

Warshowsky, J.H. (1996) "Warshowsky Stop 'n Go Free Space Fusion Trainer." *Journal of Behavioral Optometry 7*, 1, 3–4.

Warshowsky, J.H. (1996) "Ego Duality – A Mind/Body Experience." *Journal of Optometric Vision Development 27*, 4, 220–223.

Warshowsky, J.H. with FitzGerald, D.E. (1999) "Behavioral Attributes of a Low Plus Vertical Yoked Prism Correction: A Case Study." *Journal of Optometric Vision Development 30*, 4, 181–187.

Warshowsky, J.H. (2001) "Critical Empathy Revisited." *Journal of Optometric Vision Development 32*, 4, 22–25.

Warshowsky, J.H. (2008) "Vergence as a Self Perception Relationship Function." *Journal of Behavioral Optometry 19*, 6, 151–154.

Weinstein, M. (1967) "A Rational of Vision and Visual Behavior." *Journal of the American Optometric Association 38*, 12, 1030.

Glossary

(ocular) Accommodation

A unit adjustment of the eye to obtain maximal sharpness of the retinal image of an object of regard; the changes in the crystalline lens of the eye to gain a clear focus.

Accommodative esotropia

The over-crossing of the eyes due to an excessive amount of focusing.

Amblyopia

The inability to correct visual acuity even with the appropriate lens correction.

Anisometropia

A significant difference in refractive error between two eyes (i.e., optical prescription of the two eyes).

Astigmatism

An optical defect causing blurred vision because of an irregularity in an optical surface.

Awareness

The ability to have perception or knowledge.

Balance

A state of equilibrium between opposing forces (e.g. body movement against gravity).

Behavioral optometrist

The behavioral optometrist prescribes lenses, prisms, and vision therapy programs in order to prevent visual dysfunction, alleviate visual problems, and enhance visual performance by means guided by understanding the concept of vision: that vision involves the whole body within the visual process, that visual dysfunction is preventable, and that the etiology of a visual problem is developmental or induced by visual stress.

Binocular
The use of both eyes simultaneously in such a manner that each retinal image contributes to the final percept.

Centering
An awareness of body and position in space, relative to objects within that space, generated by convergence.

Convergence
The simultaneous turning inward of two eyes to one point.

Development
An orderly, sequential, chronological process characterized by (1) maturation of stature (anatomy of the individual), (2) sequential emergence of function (physiological, voluntary, and involuntary use of maturing structures and refinement of performances) and (3) interaction with the environment.

Disequilibrium
A loss of equilibrium.

Divergence
The turning outward of the two eyes.

Dysfunction
Abnormal imperfect functioning.

Egocentric process
A process whereby one knows one's position in space relative to an object in that space.

Equilibrium
A state of balance between two opposing actions or forces.

Esotropia
A condition when one eye points inward separate from the other.

Exotropia

A condition when one eye points outward separate from the other.

Farsightedness

An optical defect that causes distant objects to be seen more easily than near objects; visual images focus behind the retina.

Fixation

The process, condition, or act of directing the eye toward the object of regard causing, in a normal eye, the image of the object to be centered on the fovea.

Functional amblyopia

The inability to correct visual acuity even with the appropriate lens correction based on non-physical or non-organic conditions (i.e., not related to disease or physical manifestations other than refractive error and eye muscle imbalance).

Fusion

The act or process of blending, uniting, or cohering. In vision, the process by which a single cortical image is perceived as a result of two separate ocular ones.

Gravitational insecurity

Poor sensory modulation of vestibular function as they relate to function and proprioceptive input manifested by movement; an irrational fear of movement.

Gross motor function

A process by which a muscle or set of muscles is innervated which causes a limb or set of limbs to move.

Hypertropia

Strabismus characterized by the upward deviation of the line of sight of the non-fixating eye with reference to that of the fixating eye.

Identification

The capability to find, retrieve, report, change, or delete specific data without ambiguity, generated by accommodation.

Illusion

A misleading image presented to one's vision, a mistaken idea, misapprehension, misconception, fancy.

Image

A mental picture or conception.

In-coordination

The inability to coordinate voluntary muscular movements.

Integration

The pulling together and organizing of all of the motor stimuli that are impinging on the organism at a given moment.

Kinesthetic

A sense mediated by nervous elements in muscles, tendons, and joints, and stimulated by body movements and tension.

Midline

The center of the body going from head to toe.

Monocular

The use of one eye while the other eye is shut or covered.

Motor analog of fusion

This represents the physical lining up of the two eyes, which is necessary for the sensory component of depth perception.

Near point of convergence

The point of intersection of the lines of sight when the eyes are in the position of maximum convergence.

Nearsightedness

An optical defect that enables near objects to be seen more easily than far objects; visual images focus in front of the retina.

Perception

The mechanism whereby the organism or intellect recognizes a stimulus and makes sense out of it so that it can be utilized by the integrative system.

Position in space

The direct awareness of the spatial properties of an object, especially in relation to the observer.

Posture

The relative arrangement of the different parts of the body; the position or bearing of the body as a whole.

Proprioception

A sense of the relative position of the body and resultant movement.

Refractive error

An eyeglass prescription consisting of nearsightedness, farsightedness, and/or astigmatism.

Retina

The sensory membrane lining the inner eye, used to receive an image.

Rhythm

The flow of movement to time.

Self

The essential person separate from all other persons; identity.

Sensory motor

The integration of sensory and motor processing.

Strabismus

A condition where both eyes do not point at the same place at the same time.

Spatial organization

The arrangement or constitution of interdependent parts in space.

Spatial relationships

The connection of interdependent parts in space.

Suppression

The turning off of one eye in favor of the other during conflict of eye coordination.

Vestibular

The sensory system that responds to changes in head and body movement in space, and which coordinates eyes, head, and body.

Vision

The sense by which objects, their form, color, position, etc. in the external environment are perceived by the stimulation of light.

Vision therapy

This refers to the arranging of conditions whereby a child or adult may learn adequate degrees of freedom of movement to permit efficient visual functioning for the interpretation of light energy patterns.

Visual acuity

To look at, to see, the measurements of the threshold of discrimination of the smallest letters or symbols seen at a specific viewing distance. The ratio 20/20 refers to average sight at 20 feet. The top number represents the distance a person being tested stands from the eye chart. The bottom number represents how far away a person with normal vision can be from the chart and still read the letters in that line. A person with normal vision can read the 20/20 line from 20 feet away, the 20/200 line from 200 feet away, and the 20/10 line from 10 feet away.

Visual integration

The ability to perceive and interpret what the eyes see.

Index